THE ELITE
ATHLETE

La Crosse Exercise and Health Series

Philip K. Wilson, EdD, Series Editor
Executive Director
La Crosse Exercise Program
University of Wisconsin-La Crosse

Epidemiology, Behavior Change, and Intervention in Chronic Disease, edited by Linda K. Hall, PhD; and G. Curt Meyer, MS

Evaluation and Management of Eating Disorders: Anorexia, Bulimia, and Obesity, edited by Kristine Clark, MS, RD; Richard Parr, EdD; and William Castelli, MD

Cardiac Rehabilitation: Exercise Testing and Prescription, Volume II, edited by Linda K. Hall, PhD; and G. Curt Meyer, MS

Cardiac Rehabilitation: Exercise Testing and Prescription*, edited by Linda K. Hall, PhD; G. Curt Meyer, MS; and Herman K. Hellerstein, MD

Evaluation and Treatment of Obesity*, edited by Jean Storlie, MS, RD; and Henry A. Jordan, MD

Behavioral Management of Obesity*, edited by Jean Storlie, MS, RD; and Henry A. Jordan, MD

Nutrition and Exercise in Obesity Management*, edited by Jean Storlie, MS, RD; and Henry A. Jordan, MD

The Elite Athlete*, edited by Nancy K. Butts, PhD; Thomas T. Gushiken, PhD; and Bertram Zarins, MD

*These five books were part of the Sports Medicine and Health Science series originally published by Spectrum Publications. Henry S. Miller, MD, served as the associate series editor.

THE ELITE ATHLETE

Edited by

Nancy K. Butts, PhD
Thomas T. Gushiken, PhD
University of Wisconsin-La Crosse
La Crosse, Wisconsin

Bertram Zarins, MD
Massachusetts General Hospital
Boston, Massachusetts

Life Enhancement Publications
Champaign, Illinois

The Elite Athlete

Library of Congress Cataloging-in-Publication Data

The Elite athlete.

(La Crosse exercise and health series)
Outgrowth of the Elite Athlete Tract of the 1983
La Crosse Health and Sports Science Symposium, sponsored
by the La Crosse Exercise Program of the University of
Wisconsin—La Crosse.
Reprint. Originally published: New York : SP Medical
& Scientific Books, c1985. Originally published in series:
Sports medicine and health science.
Includes bibliographies and index.
1. Sports medicine. 2. Sports—Physiological aspects.
3. Sports—Psychological aspects. 4. Human mechanics.
5. Sports sciences. I. Butts, Nancy K. (Nancy Kay)
II. Gushiken, Thomas T. III. Zarins, Bertram.
IV. La Crosse Health and Sports Science Symposium
(1983). Elite Athlete Tract. V. La Crosse Exercise
Program (University of Wisconsin—La Crosse) VI. Series.
[DNLM: 1. Biomechanics—congresses. 2. Sports—con-
gresses. 3. Sports Medicine—congresses.
QT 260 E43 1983a]
RC1210.E43 1987   617'.1027   87-22860
ISBN 0-87322-905-3

ISSN 0894-4261
ISBN 0-87322-905-3

Printed in the United States of America

10 9 8 7 6 5 4 3 2 1

Life Enhancement Publications
A Division of Human Kinetics Publishers, Inc.
Box 5076, Champaign, IL 61820
1-800-DIAL-HKP
1-800-334-3665 (in Illinois)

Contributors

Patrick W. Bradley, Ph.D.   Department of Sports Physiology, Sports Medicine Division, U.S. Olympic Committee, Colorado Springs, Colorado

Nancy Kay Butts, Ph.D.   Director, Research Unit, LaCrosse Exercise Program; Professor of Physical Education, University of Wisconsin-LaCrosse

Kenneth S. Clarke, Ph.D.   Director, Sports Medicine and Science Division, U.S. Olympic Committee, Colorado Springs, Colorado

Denise Daily-McKee, M.D.   Resident, Family and Community Medicine, School of Medicine, University of Nevada-Reno

Charles J. Dillman, Ph.D.   Director, Sports Science Department, Sports Medicine Division, U.S. Olympic Committee, Colorado Springs, Colorado

Keith French, Ph.D.   Chairman, Department of Physical Education; Director, Biomechanics Laboratory, University of Wisconsin-LaCrosse

George Furman, M.D.   Professor, Obstetrics and Gynecology, School of Medicine, University of Nevada-Reno

Ann C. Grandjean, M.S., R.D.   Nutrition Consultant, U.S. Olympic Committee, Sports Medicine Division; Associate Director, Swanson Center for Nutrition, Omaha, Nebraska

Thomas T. Gushiken, Ph.D. Director, Workshop-Symposium Unit, LaCrosse Exercise Program; Associate Professor, Department of Recreation, University of Wisconsin-LaCrosse

Sandra J. Harms, M.S. Department of Sports Physiology, Sports Medicine Division, U.S. Olympic Committee, Colorado Springs, Colorado

Dorothy Harris, Ph.D. Sports Psychology Advisory Committee, U.S. Olympic Committee; Coordinator of Graduate Program in Sports Psychology, Pennsylvania State University, University Park

Michael W. Herring, B.S. Statistician, Office of Evaluation and Educational Research, School of Medicine, University of Nevada-Reno

Ralph Mann, Ph.D. Director, Biomechanics Laboratory, Compu-Sport, Ocala, Florida

Jerry R. May, Ph.D. Co-Chairman, Sports Psychology Committee, U.S. Olympic Committee; Associate Professor of Psychiatry and Behavioral Sciences, Department of Psychiatry and Behavioral Science, School of Medicine, University of Nevada-Reno

William Nelson, M.S. Biomechanical Research Consultant, U.S. Olympic Committee and U.S. Rowing Association; Mechanical Engineer, Crown Center Redevelopment Corp., Kansas City, Missouri

Mary Margaret Newsom, M.S. Department of Education Services, Sports Medicine Division, U.S. Olympic Committee, Colorado Springs, Colorado

Richard B. Parr, Ed.D. Professor and Co-Director of Health Fitness Program, Central Michigan University, Mt. Pleasant

Michael L. Pollock, Ph.D. Director, Cardiac Rehabilitation and Human Performance Laboratory, Universal Services Rehabilitation and Development, Inc., Houston, Texas

Jackie L. Puhl, Ph.D. Department of Sports Physiology, Sports Medicine Division, U.S. Olympic Committee, Colorado Springs, Colorado

Scott W. Southard, M.D. Department of Orthopedic Surgery, Maricopa County General Hospital, Phoenix, Arizona

Peter J. Van Handel, Ph.D. Department of Sports Physiology, Sports Medicine Division, U.S. Olympic Committee, Colorado Springs, Colorado

Tracy L. Veach, Ed.D. Assistant Professor, Psychiatry and Behavioral Sciences, School of Medicine, University of Nevada-Reno

Luther L. Williams, M.S. Pike's Peak Diagnostic Laboratory, Colorado Springs, Colorado

Bertram Zarins, M.D. Chairman, Education Committee, U.S. Olympic Committee, Sports Medicine Council; Head Physician, U.S. Olympic Team (1984 Winter Olympics); Assistant Clinical Professor of Orthopaedic Surgery, Harvard Medical School; Chief of Sports Medicine Unit, Massachusetts General Hospital; Team Physician, New England Patriots and Boston Bruins

Contents

I. Administration

II. Biomechanics

III. Psychology of Sports

Contents

IV. Physiology

V. Nutrition

Afterword

Preface

It is with great pleasure that we present *The Elite Athlete* for use as a reference and/or textbook. This text is an outgrowth of The Elite Athlete Tract of the 1983 La Crosse Health and Sports Science Symposium, sponsored annually by the La Crosse Exercise Program of the University of Wisconsin–La Crosse. The elite athlete topic was chosen as one of the four tracts of the 1983 symposium due to the timeliness of the 1984 Winter and Summer Olympic Games. The versatility of the authors and their topics contributed to an exciting symposium—and now, an exciting book.

It is appropriate that the Foreword of this book be written by Dr. Bertram Zarins, Chairman of the Education Committee of the U.S. Olympic Sports Medicine Council. No one knows better the problems, needs, and future directions of the medical aspects of the elite athlete than Dr. Zarins. It is equally fitting that the Administrative Section involve Dr. Clark and Ms. Newsom, as again their assignments with the U.S. Olympic Committee provide a unique perspective on the administrative aspects of the elite athlete. Sections II through V cover the areas of biomechanics, psychology, physiology, and nutrition, which are essential components in the development of the elite athlete. The book concludes with an Afterword, a most revealing discussion of the elite athlete at the Masters level.

The editors and individual chapter authors of this book should be complimented for providing an exciting, interesting, and valuable book. It is hoped this book will provide intellectual as well as enjoyable reading to all associated with the elite athlete, and most importantly will provide additional insights and directions to assist in the future development of the elite athlete.

Philip K. Wilson, Ed.D., Senior Series Editor
Henry S. Miller, M.D., Associate Series Editor

Foreword

CHALLENGE TO SPORTS MEDICINE
IN THE UNITED STATES

Bertram Zarins

The IX Pan American Games held in Caracas, Venezuela, in August 1983 will be remembered for its drug scandal. Eleven athletes were disqualified because traces of banned drugs were found in their urine specimens. Twelve U.S athletes dropped out of competition and flew home, and others either developed injuries or performed well below their expected levels. Public criticism was directed mainly toward the athletes. This crisis should sound a warning note to all of us involved in sports medicine: the drug issue presents a major challenge to sports medicine today.

A question we should ask ourselves is whether the athletes are the ones to blame fully for taking drugs. Why did the athletes violate moral, ethical, and legal standards at the expense of their own health to try to improve performance? Did we fail in identifying and in meeting the needs of the elite athlete? Should we not strive to provide better and safer ways of improving performance than drugs? How can we redirect our energies to better meet the goals of the elite athlete?

As we approach the end of each Olympic quadrennium and look forward to the next, we should pause to reflect on our activities in the field of sports medicine to see if we are on course. I would like to take an overview of the relatively new field of sports medicine, to examine the progress we have made to date and to look at the work that still needs to be done. In analyzing the challenges facing us today, I break the task down into three components:

1. What are the *goals* and *needs* of the elite athlete?
2. How can we channel our activities to help them meet their needs and reach their goals?
3. How can we *cooperate* with one another to combine our resources and prevent duplication in meeting these goals?

Let us look at these three components separately.

IDENTIFYING THE GOALS AND NEEDS OF THE ELITE ATHLETE

The *goal* of the elite athlete is to perform at the very highest possible level. Athletes may have the natural ability to do so, but they probably need the help of coaches, trainers, physicians, or other scientists to reach this goal. Athletes would like to avoid injury. If injured, they would like to have proper medical diagnosis and treatment and return to their sports as quickly as possible.

Successful individuals, including athletes, usually have clear-cut goals and work purposefully in meeting these goals. The same is true for successful corporations: All those working for the company know their own goals and those of the corporation. Less effective individuals or organizations often lack clear-cut goals or objectives. They tend to be activity oriented rather than goal oriented. Another way to put it is: "If you don't know where you're going, any road will do."

The athlete and coach should know the goals and needs in a sport better than anyone else. Communication among athlete, coach, and scientist is essential. Athletes and coaches must provide the problems to be solved. When science or medicine comes up with answers, these must be explained to the athlete and coach so they can be implemented. All too often, a scientist carries out an experiment and comes up with answers to a question that is not pertinent to the needs of athlete, or useful information rests in the library because the athlete and coach do not know how to interpret or implement the data.

DIRECTING OUR ACTIVITIES AND RESOURCES TO MEET THE NEEDS OF ATHLETES IN REACHING THEIR GOALS

Let us look at various activities in the field of sports medicine to see how they measure up to the test of being goal oriented and where changes need to be made.

Research and Application of Scientific Principles

Perhaps the greatest impact in the development of an elite athlete program can be made in the areas of screening and selection of athletes. What are the physical and mental characteristics that allow an individual to excel in a sport? How can these characteristics be identified at an early age? How can children be directed toward sports in which they have the potential of becoming elite?

Considerable scientific and clinical research is being applied toward physical conditioning with the goal of improving performance. Some of this time is being spent in areas of physiology which yield little results. Testing of athletes tends to be fragmentary with little follow-up or implementation. For example, a single determination of anerobic threshold, $\dot{V}O_2$ max, or muscle fiber type may help in the publication of a scientific paper but rarely helps the athlete or coach.

Research in the field of ergogenic aids and drugs has largely been taboo in the United States while it reportedly is common in certain other countries. Athletes in certain sports, such as weight lifting, believe they cannot win without drugs. They are left to their own devices since we turn our backs to them. We must develop alternatives to improving performance without the use of ergogenic aids which will be more attractive to the elite athlete than drugs.

Athletes need to apply proper biomechanical principles if they are to achieve superior results. They must understand forces, velocities, vectors, and other physical principles. Coaches should be even more knowledgeable in this area to properly advise the athlete. This knowledge should extend to playing surfaces, shoes, and protective and other equipment.

Biomechanical analysis of performance is being used to an increasing extent. Techniques such as three dimensional motion analysis and formation analysis are gaining popularity as the tools become available. As with physiological testing, these data are scientifically interesting but of little use to the athlete or coach unless they can be applied.

A real need exists for sport specific research. Each sport has its unique demands and problems, and these must be identified and studied. To help meet this need, the American Orthopaedic Society for Sports Medicine has undertaken a major research study into injuries in certain sports. The United States Olympic Committee (USOC) and National Governing Bodies are cooperating in this study, which will be expanded to include more sports.

Medical Care

The quality of medical care and level of science and technology supporting medicine in the United States are among the best in the world. However, there are countries with lower levels of medical care and science that mobilize a greater degree of medical support for their athletes. One of the things we must do is direct a greater percentage of our medical resources toward meeting the needs of athletes. This does not necessarily mean the development of new resources or technology but the application of currently existing resources to improving the health and performance of our athletes. Our medical system is geared toward the treatment of injury or illness once it has occurred. We should redirect the focus toward enhancing health and preventing disease and injury.

Education

Education in the field of sports medicine for physicians and researchers is on a high level, thanks to efforts of organizations such as the American Orthopaedic Society for Sports Medicine (AOSSM) and American College of Sports Medicine (ACSM). Physical therapists and athletic trainers also have formal continuing education programs. Formal education curricula and certification for coaches are largely lacking and represent an area where considerable progress is due. Improving the knowledge of our coaches is the most direct way we can influence our athletes.

Education of the athletes themselves, of course, is the ultimate goal if we are to influence the use of ergogenic aids. We should expand our use of new communication media to reach large groups of athletes.

COOPERATING WITH ONE ANOTHER TO BETTER REACH OUR GOALS

The United States does not have a national organizational force or agency that controls sports or sports medicine. This is a reflection of our individuality and freedom. There are countries that have so much control over their people that they can clearly direct activities through well-organized machines. I do not think that most of us would want to sacrifice our freedom for control even though this could result in a more efficient means of obtaining success in international sports competition. We must achieve our goals by cooperating with one another.

In the United States the field of sports medicine is still in a state of flux. There are a number of sports medicine organizations—some old, some new, some with overlapping and some with competing spheres of influence. The American College of Sports Medicine was founded in 1955, and the American Orthopaedic Society for Sports Medicine was founded in 1973. There are more than seventy-five other national groups that deal with sports medicine.

The United States Olympic Committee had little to do with sports medicine until the Amateur Sports Act of 1978 was passed by Congress. This act placed a major responsibility on the United States Olympic Committee of establishing, coodinating, and directing policy related to amateur sports in the United States.

The United States Olympic Committee has established as its goals in the area of sports medicine to be as follows:

1. To achieve optimal health and superior performance in athletes.
2. To provide and to coordinate sports medicine services for United States teams, sports organizations, and National Governing Bodies and the United States Olympic Committee.
3. To promote the benefits of Olympic sports medicine and Olympic ideals for all.

Despite this act of Congress, there is no real organized control of sports medicine in the United States. Unification may never occur because of the nature of our system. Therefore, mutual cooperation is the way we have to proceed at this time. This may be the greatest challenge facing us in this decade.

I have seen recent changes in the attitudes of various sports medicine organizations in the United States from one of fierce individualism to an attitude that is less defensive and more inclined to cooperate with other organizations. In May 1982, the American Medical Association hosted a two-day meeting for sports and medical organizations in the United States that deal with sports medicine. Subsequently, meetings have been held between the ACSM, USOC, AOSSM, NATA and the President's Council on Physical Fitness and Sports to see how these organizations can work together. The AOSSM is undertaking an ambitious project of sport-specific analysis into causes and prevention of injury in cooperation with other organizations. In the area of education, we are seeing more conferences held jointly.

The issue of anabolic steroids and other ergogenic aids deserve special mention. Our society is known for excess drug use, so it is not really surprising that athletes take drugs. We are not surprised that they take excessive vitamins or shocked if they use mind-altering drugs. The issue of using drugs to improve performance is more controversial and serious. Some drugs are taken for their psychologic effect to gain an "edge" on the opponent; others are taken to add body weight and muscle mass artificially.

There are four approaches one might take in dealing with the problem of ergogenic aids in sports: (1) ignore the problem, (2) detect and punish, (3) assist users to minimize harmful effects of the drugs they are taking and, (4) provide the athlete with better alternatives than drugs.

The USOC has taken a firm stand on the issue of doping and chose a program of detection and enforcement of regulations together with a research program to find better alternatives.

SUMMARY

The field of sports medicine in the United States is in a process of evolution. It is an exciting time to be involved in sports medicine since changes are taking place rapidly and we are in a position to affect these changes. I must stress our most important challenge: we must not lose sight of our purpose for being in sports medicine—to meet the needs of the athlete. We must remain *goal* oriented and not *activity* oriented.

Finally, we should be sure our sports organizations, medical societies, and sports medicine groups cooperate with one another in sharing information and pooling resources. Memberships may be different, but there is a common goal that should not be forgotten.

As we move toward the end of this Olympic quadrennium and the pinnacle of amateur athletics, the Olympiad, we should look at the elite athlete, striving to achieve the best performance humanly possible. This individual has devoted years to intense training and has spared nothing in his or her quest to be the best in the world. We should do everything possible to help the athlete in the pursuit of excellence.

I.
Administration

CHAPTER 1

The United States Olympic Committee Sports Medicine Program: An Overview

Kenneth S. Clarke

The elite athlete is a specimen of mankind that is unique in many ways from the rest of us and one that is primarily redundant with us in other ways. The challenge of an elite athlete sports medicine program is not merely, "How do I attend to thee, let me count the ways,". but also "Which way, which way, that is the question," with "which way" referring both to the selection of attentions that have the best chance of helping an elite athlete be more elite and the selection of a logistical system that delivers these attentions to these athletes within the realities of our society.

Sports medicine, for the sake of this chapter, consequently is the sum of attentions experienced by an athlete that supports his/her pursuit of excellence. These attentions may be clinical, both as to the preventive and remedial goals of the practitioner, and they may be conceptual, both as to evaluative and applicative goals of the scientist. But they remain the experience of the athlete.

Based in part on Clarke, K., "The Amateur Sports Act of 1978—Implications for Sports Medicine," *Symposium on Olympic Sports Medicine*. W. B. Saunders, 1983, pp. 7-12.

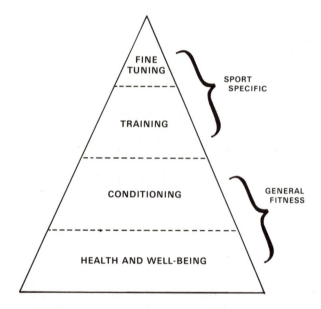

Figure 1.1. Sports medicine in perspective.

The triangle model in Figure 1.1 depicts the focus of sports medicine attentions to that end. As in sports, fundamentals and special skills are involved. The base is the *health and well-being* of the person; it is difficult to "peak" with an abscessed tooth or an emotional concern. *Conditioning* produces the general fitness for activity that all should seek, while *training* constitutes the hard work directed toward handling the particular strength and endurance requirements of a given sport. *Fine tuning* is what separates athletes of equivalent skill and training—getting the extra edge reliably (consistently) through an athlete's fullest "reading" and use of his/her body's resources for that sport at the time of competition.

None of this is done by merely defining sports medicine. It is done by linking the resources of the scientist, the judgment of the clinician, and the motivation and talent of the athlete with the strategy and perception of the coach. The United States Olympic Committee (USOC) Sports Medicine Division is now building those linkages. In most countries it is relatively easy to "bunch" the above people by fiat, by direct order. In our society, it must happen through logistical expertise, altruism, and national respect for the commitment of the amateur athlete to personal excellence.

In November 1978, Congress passed and President Carter signed into Law PL 95-606, which modified the charter of the USOC and concluded officially a long chapter of controversy among sports governance bodies over the control of competitions for the nation's elite athletes. With the enactment of this act, the Amateur Sports Act of 1978, USOC was given a clear mandate and foundation for being a unifying force in amateur athletics—i.e., assisting national governing bodies (NGBs) who by that Act were given responsibility for developing the respective Olympic sports in this country while respecting the prerogatives of sports organizations who restrict competition to specific classes of athletes (e.g., National Collegiate Athletic Association and college students).

A number of the features of the Act (such as, arbitration procedures for complaints) had already been adopted by USOC constitutional amendment a few years earlier. Nonetheless, extensive constitutional changes followed to clarify as well as to broaden the scope of USOC's attentions consistent with the enacted law. Included among the new features were increased representation of athletes in the governance process (20% of all committees and the House of Delegates); affirmative commitment to the participation of the handicapped, women, and minorities; and expressed commitment to the implementation of sports medicine concepts and practices on behalf of all amateur athletes.

The immediate result of this legislative action was a reorganization of the USOC itself accompanied by a profound shift in budgetary goals that would support the minimum expectations from the Amateur Sports Act. The change from suiting, transporting, and feeding our Olympic athletes to developing greater opportunity for Olympic hopefuls to pursue as well as to achieve is indeed worthy of the description "profound," going from a quadrennial budget of $14.8 million in 1973-1976 to $80.1 million for 1981-1984. With the U.S. being essentially the only one of the 150 countries in the Olympics that does not receive subsidy from its federal government, the Amateur Sports Act forced both the necessity of new budget levels and new programs that would reflect credibility to the public and corporations who must be approached to contribute dollars voluntarily to this extent and to our professional colleagues in sports medicine who enable us to extend attentions to the athletes.

ORGANIZATIONAL JURISDICTION

At this point, it is necessary to clarify the respective organizational "turfs" of USOC, the NGBs, and the Los Angeles Olympic Organizing Committee (LAOOC). The LAOOC was the organization franchised by the International Olympic Committee (IOC) to stage the 1984 Summer Games on behalf of all participating countries. It was their task to prepare the housing, athletic, and medical facilities and the logistics that must accompany them. Their budget and fund-raising structure were delimited to that task force goal of "pulling it off." Sarajevo, Yugoslavia, has its local organizing committee as well with identical tasks, but not being in the United States, it did not cause the confusions relative to USOC as does LAOOC.

The NGBs, on the other hand, respectively are responsible for the development of their sports in continuous manner throughout the quadrennium, including the identification through due process of the athletes who have earned the right to represent the U.S. in international competition. Their respective budgets are autonomous, self-determined by perceived goal and resource, and in turn self-determine the extensiveness of their ability to develop their sport. Collectively, the NGBs have 51% of the vote in USOC's House of Delegates.

The USOC assumes jurisdiction over the respective NGBs through review/approval of their procedures for selecting their international delegation and subsequently the management of the collective U.S. teams at the Olympic and Pan American Games, the World University Games, and the National Sports Festivals. The USOC assumes further responsibility for the special resources it provides to NGBs who elect to utilize these resources—e.g., development grants and the Olympic Training Center. USOC resources thereby are separate from both the NGBs and the LAOOC, yet related to both. The USOC must take the best of whatever athletes the NGB can provide for the Olympic Games and experience the best of whatever the local Olympic organizing committee can muster to conduct the games. The advantages of cooperative efforts within prerogative are clear. The better the USOC can assist NGBs and local Olympic organizing committees and vice versa, the better all can fulfill their objectives, especially with respect to sports medicine.

USOC AND SPORTS MEDICINE

The sports medicine program has paralleled the changes in USOC, striving to be a unifying force in this field of attention on behalf of amateur athletes. In its first full quadrennium, its budget is nearly equal to that for all of USOC except four Olympiads earlier, yet still somewhat austere considering the missions involved. Combined with the Sports Medicine Council, the official policy-formulating, direction-steering body appointed by the USOC President for the quadrennium composed of volunteers of diverse expertise, is the Sports Medicine Division, the professional support staff component that conducts and extends approved programs. Both the Council and the Division recognize that whatever is conducted should be extended in a manner that both sets a standard of quality and nature for NGBs to emulate and also fosters assistance to NGB volunteers and employed staff. Because of the glamourous mystique of sports medicine, however, many things are promoted, justified, and experienced in its name, and the outer boundaries of legitimacy are mighty jagged. The USOC Sports Medicine Program, therefore, must be assisted by quality volunteer colleagues in the field, to help all 38 national sports governing bodies reach their athletes with some logic and order.

The Division's structural organization is designed as the nerve center for these operations. It reflects the planning of the "original" Sports Medicine Council (i.e., the council in office at the time of the Amateur Sports Act) and includes the refinements of the 1981–1984 council to embark on an ambitious pursuit of a balance in service, research, and education throughout the quadrennium. Clinical services remains a fundamental department (the Clinical Services Department), now expanded to include dental- and vision-screening programs. Receiving new and equivalent significance are the Sports Physiology, Biomechanics, and Education Services Departments.

With time, budget, and greater familiarity with policy implementation nuances, each of these staff attentions have their counterpart within the Council through its standing committees. Between the council chairman and the division director, consequently the best of both segments of the USOC sports medicine program are guided into an integrated operation.

Clinical Services

The two basic missions of this department and its companion Medical Committee of the Council are to provide competent medical attentions to athletes (1) at the Olympic Training Center (OTC) and (2) at the competitive events for which USOC has responsibility (i.e., National Sports Festivals, World University Games, Pan American Games, and Olympic Games). The two missions are interdependent. With a daily presence of 200–700 athletes at the OTC representing any of 38 sports, the cost of an accompanying employed medical staff would be prohibitive. In practice, one physician and two certified athletic trainers are employed with the remaining staff coming to OTC out of application for volunteer service. Criteria include five years minimum experience with varsity-level athletes with preference given to physicians or certified athletic trainers with demonstrated excellent service to an NGB.

OTC service as a volunteer, on the other hand, is a prerequisite to eligibility for consideration as a nominee to the Pan American and Olympic teams' medical staffs. The reason is that medical attention to elite athletes in those scenarios is much different from that experienced by either a high-school or college team physician or a practitioner at a sports medicine clinic. The clinical significance of a complaint must be assessed under field conditions and the intensity of world-class competition away from one's customary staff and equipment. The resulting management must be either to refer (to the local games committee medical resources or back home) or to disqualify the athlete if the assessment discerned a malady of significance, or either to condone or prescribe appropriate proprietary management in the attempt to return the stricken athlete to participation. Further, this is done with limited previous knowledge of the athlete and potentially of the sports in which he/she is competing, and with the assistance of colleagues whom one may have just met.

The IOC places quotas on the size of a team's medical staff (e.g., 8 at the Winter Olympics and 24 at the Summer Olympics). Within that figure must be the entire array of physicians, athletic trainers, and any other type of practitioner (e.g., dentist, psychologist) a country wishes to send. Consequently, there is no possible way for sport "specialists" (e.g., a physician with experience only with judo athletes) to be selected for the U.S. medical staffs. To entrust our nation's elite athletes to these decisions requires advance experience under similar conditions and evaluation of those experiences. The OTC is an ideal proving ground for such. The subsequent assignment at a sports festival adds the touch of the real thing— sole attention on competition.

Clinical services at OTC, however, are not limited to the diagnosis, treatment, and short-term rehabilitation of customary injuries and illnesses. Vision and dental screening programs, for example, are conducted to enable preventive and enhancing services to be applied.

Research and Evaluation

The commitment to evaluate both the athlete and principles related to performance enhancement is a new opportunity for USOC subsequent to the Amateur Sports Act. The USOC operating budget does not yet permit "requests for proposals" for research protocols from research laboratories/clinics on a competitive basis, but it does permit both the development of staff-coordinated laboratories at OTC (sports physiology, biomechanics) and evaluated experiences with linking these resources with the resources of others in the field for expanded pursuits of common goals.

Customary research has the scientist preconceiving the curiosity and developing the strict protocol to be followed to satisfy the curiosity with disinterested objectivity—i.e., the athletes come to the scientist, and deductions are made for application to the athlete who is similar to the subjects tested. In contrast, the expedience of the Olympic moment gives priority for USOC staff to meet the curiosities of the elite athlete (in essence, how am I compared to myself, or theoretical model of perfection, or the best athlete in my sport, and how can I improve), and the scientist must create a protocol that brings objectivity and meaning to the exercise—i.e., the scientist comes to the athlete, and feedback must be immediate and relevant. Inductive relevance for the athlete population of that sport is examined as well if the individuals' data are poolable. Ideally, both approaches to new information and its application should be supported and integrated, and both the USOC Sports Medicine Council and Division are devoted to these ends. In fact, our budding network of biomechanists and exercise physiologists are rapidly demonstrating the value of this approach to our athletes and coaches.

Education

The Amateur Sports Act reflects strongly the expectation to disseminate the current state-of-the-art sports medicine concepts and practices to various target populations. As a unifying force, USOC stands to benefit from assisting allied institutions and organizations with the capability for such, as well as conducting selected programs of their own if not otherwise available. These programs include workshops for invited experts to arrive at new knowledge and/or concensus on prevailing issues (chronobiology, boxing safety, chiropractic), conferences for special groups utilizing selected experts as the faculty (modalities, nutrition, sport psychology), correspondence and audiovisual materials in response to requests for information, and information-retrieval system and other clearinghouse functions for referring inquirers to sources of the information requested. All such programs are receiving organized attentions at USOC and through increased organizational liaison with national organizations having related missions.

SPECIAL NOTES

These four areas, clinical, physiology, biomechanics, and education serve as departmental and committee homes for whatever activities acknowledge the original sports medicine premise that human performance is of a complex mosaic nature. Some interest areas that are either too specific or too interdisciplinary to warrant department status (e.g., nutrition, weight training, sports psychology, and safety attentions) are either woven into the existing services or are launched as special projects with assimilation determined by the experience gained. For example, USOC now has a standing committee on Sports Equipment and Technology so that the special expertise needed to produce better bobsleds and bikes, safer equipment, and garb, etc., can be organized.

Further, too few appreciate that our nation's elite athletes who compete internationally include some who do so in wheelchairs or with sight or hearing disability—i.e., the so-called "handicapped." These customarily atypical considerations are now becoming customary and typical within USOC's support system for sports medicine. The USOC Committee on Sports for the Disabled works closely with the Sports Medicine Council for the extension of quality sports medicine attentions to these athletes, with implications for adaptations coming from evaluation and study, not merely tradition and that bane of progress, "common sense."

The last special project I will mention is the Elite Athlete Project that was launched in January 1982 to gain needed experience in reaching and assisting the elite athletes within the tenets of our society. Four administrative goals of integration were established: (1) to help the NGBs develop their cadre of interdisciplinary sports medicine leadership, (2) to share USOC expertise and resources, (3) to credential and link research resources in the field with clusters of athletes, (4) and to pilot some broad-based basic research with generic applicative value. To accomplish these goals, it takes time to establish the rapport to determine how to work together; it takes feedback that is immediately applicable and evaluated; it takes a network of expertise for responding meaningfully to special concerns, whether it be drugs or hemorrhoids or chronobiology; and it takes a perspective for learning which of the sports medicine attentions are transferrable to other elite athletes, developing elite athletes, and/or all active persons in the United States.

Sports medicine, consequently, is a support service of vital significance to the Olympic ideals. It does not produce medals; it supports athletes who have the motivation through sport to pursue excellence and the other benefits of an active life. The United States Olympic Committee deeply appreciates the many contributions of equipment, supplies, and funds by so many corporations, and the contributions of altruistic service by so many colleagues in the field to provide an effective Olympic sports medicine program to our nation's athlete hopefuls.

CHAPTER 2

A Brief Introduction to Information Retrieval for the Sports Medicine Practitioner

Mary Margaret Newsom

Some libraries provide online search services at no charge to their patrons, but others must of necessity charge for the actual costs of computer connect time and/or a service charge. Costs for use of online databases can vary anywhere from $15 per hour to $200 per hour or higher, so again, knowledge of the contents of the databases and understanding of their use is most important. During recent years, the increasingly widespread use of home computers has also meant the use of online databases by an increasing number of home users, though for many the cost may be prohibitive.

The search process usually begins with an "interview" between the requester and the information specialist to be sure there is a clear understanding of what is being sought and why. The information specialist then develops a "search strategy," or plan/map for how the database(s) will be queried to retrieve the desired information. The search itself is begun by accessing the vendor's computer via telephone connect, selecting the appropriate database, and typing the search terms (subject keywords, author name, title words, etc.). The computer searches for the occurrence of the term(s) in the selected

The Elite Athlete, edited by N. K. Butts, T. T. Gushiken, and B. Zarins. Copyright © 1985 by Spectrum Publications, Inc.

database and indicates how many citations were found. The searcher can then examine the citations (or portions thereof; for example, titles only could be listed), and can order a printout of those which are appropriate. Sometimes, if time and funds permit, it is desirable to search several databases for the same topic, since relevant information—particularly for the fields of sports medicine—can be scattered across many databases.

Once appropriate citations have been retrieved, copies of needed source document must be located. All major vendors provide online document ordering services, but such services can be quite expensive; thus, most patrons must rely on their own library's resources or interlibrary loan networks to obtain copies of source documents.

MAJOR DATABASES RELEVANT TO SPORTS MEDICINE

The question of sports medicine databases is a surprisingly difficult question to answer because sports medicine information is widely scattered across a number of databases. The decision must be made based on knowledge of what databases are available, according to how much time and money are available for searching, and how in-depth the information needs to be. Some of the relevant databases available through commercial vendors are listed in Table 2.1; for the sake of brevity, descriptions of most of these databases are not repeated here. Instead, some of the major databases which this author has found to be most helpful, as well as some important printed indexes and specialized databases, are briefly described.

SPORT Database

The largest and most comprehensive database devoted to sports science in the world is the SPORT database produced by the Coaching Association of Canada's Information Resource Center (SIRC). Begun 1973, it includes some material that dates back to the 1940s. As of December 1983, SPORT contained citations of over 90,000 documents relevant to sports in general, including physical education, recreation, physical fitness, and sports medicine. Every two months, some 3,000 citations are added to the database, from over 800 relevant journals and serials as well as from appropriate proceedings and monographs. Since 1981, SIRC has included input from the Federal Institute for Sports Science in West Germany, including German language material from Switzerland, Australia, and East Germany as well as West Germany.

SIRC/SPORT have received international acclaim from the International Association for Sport Information (IASI) and the International Council for Sport and Physical Education (ICSPE) of UNESCO and was designated in 1983 as "the" international database for sports information into which IASI member nations worldwide will provide input once negotiations are finalized and funding is settled. Through the concept proposed by IASI, the appropriate institute/organization from each member nation will coordinate documentation in that country and will then input the information into SPORT in exchange for copies of the database (in the form of magnetic tape or, in underdeveloped countries, in printed form). Currently, IASI is developing a multilingual uniform thesaurus for this use and for defining methodologies for input by member nations. The U.S. Olympic Committee has been asked to serve as coordinator for U.S.-produced information, and the feasibility and mechanism for such an arrangement are now being explored. Other countries which have expressed commitment to this international effort include Great Britain, Finland, Cuba, Mexico, East and West Germany, Bulgaria, Poland, the Netherlands, the People's Republic of China, Japan, and others.

SPORT is accessible around the world via SDC's ORBIT retrieval system; currently SIRC has an exclusive agreement with SDC, although negotiations are currently being made to make SPORT available through at least one additional vendor by early 1985. Current connect cost for access to SPORT through SDC is $85 per hour, plus telecommunications costs (which average $10 per hour). Inside Canada, searches of SPORT can be requested directly through SIRC for a considerable cost savings ($7.50 per search for the first 75 citations), but this option is not available to U.S. users.

SPORT is available in printed form via the 8-volume *Sport Bibliography*, which contains some 70,000 references to works published prior to 1980, and its 2-volume *Supplement*, which lists works published between 1980–1982. Current coverage is provided in print form via the monthly *Sport and Recreation Index*, which includes some 1,200 citations each month. Access to citations in both the bibliography and the index is by subject only, with no title access or author access; the database can be searched by multiple access points. Also the database is more likely to contain "the" most current information, due to time for production/printing of the index. However, for retrospective material, the bibliography and its

Table 2.1. Database Bibliography: Selected Listing of Databases Relevant to Sports Medicine, Available through Major Vendors (Compiled by Mary Margaret Newsom)

Database Name	Subject Area/Summary	Producer	Vendor
Biosis Preview	Biological Sciences: Includes contents of Biological Abstracts and Bioresearch Index. Contains citations from nearly 8000 primary journals, symposia, reviews, preliminary reports, semi-popular journals, selected institutional and government reports, research, communications, and other sources on all aspects of biosciences and medical research. 1969–present.	Biosciences Information Service, 2100 Arch Street, Philadelphia, PA 19103 800/523–4806	DIALOG BRS SDC
CA Search	Chemistry: Produced by the merger of CA Condensates file, which contains the basic bibliographic information appearing in the printed Chemical Abstracts, and CASIA file, which contains general subject headings from a controlled vocabulary, as well as uncontrolled vocabulary to provide users with more access points to each citation.	Chemical Abstracts Service, Columbus, OH	BRS SDC DIALOG
CHEMDEX	Chemical Dictionary files corresponding to CHEMNAME, below.		SDC
CHEMNAME	Chemistry: Listing of chemical substances in dictionary-type, nonbibliographic file; gives CAS registry number, molecular formula, CA substances index name, available synonyms, ring data, and other chemical substances data. Supports searching in CA SEARCH by specific subjects.	Chemical Abstracts Service, Columbus, OH and Lockheed DIALOG Information Retrieval Service	DIALOG
CHEMSDI	Covers information cited in the last six weeks of Chemical Abstracts; can be used as a current awareness file for both new compounds and new developments in chemistry and related fields.	Chemical Abstracts Service, Columbus, OH	SDC

Name	Description	Provider	Vendor
CHEMSEARCH	Chemistry: Dictionary, nonbibliographic listing of chemical substances recently cited in CA Search; companion file to CHEMNAME.	Lockheed DIALOG Information Retrieval Service, Palo Alto, CA	DIALOG
CIN	Chemical industry notes containing citations to business literature in the chemical industry (including pharmaceutical).	Lockheed DIALOG Information Retrieval Service, Palo Alto, CA	DIALOG
Conference Papers Index	Multidisciplinary: Contains references to scientific and technical papers presented at approximately 1000 regional, national, and international meetings; offers effective method of keeping up with ongoing research and development. Cites many research findings over a year before the findings are actually published. 1973–present.	Cambridge Scientific Abstracts, Bethesda, MD	DIALOG
Current Procedural Terminology	Contains more than 6000 descriptions of procedures and provides uniform coding and nomenclature system for reporting medical services and procedures performed by physicians.	American Medical Association, Chicago, IL	AMANET
Disease Information Base	Synopsis of over 3500 distinct disease entities, disorders, and conditions.	American Medical Association, Chicago, IL	AMANET
Dissertation Abstracts	Multidisciplinary: Definitive subject, title, and author guide to virtually every American dissertation accepted at an accredited institution since 1861; citations also included for some Canadian dissertations. (Contents correspond to Dissertation Abstracts International and American Doctoral Dissertations.)	Xerox University Microfilms, Ann Arbor, MI	BRS DIALOG
Drug Information/ Alcohol Use-Abuse	Drug and alcohol abuse.	University of Minnesota College of Pharmacy, Minneapolis, MN	BRS

(Continued)

Table 2.1. (Continued)

Database Name	Subject Area/Summary	Producer	Vendor
Drug Information Base	Evaluative information on some 1100 generic substances marked under over 5500 trade names in the U.S., Canada, Mexico.	American Medical Association, Chicago, IL	AMANET (GTE Telenet)
ERIC	Education/Multidisciplinary: Includes two main files, Research in Education, which identifies the most signficant and timely research projects, and Current Index to Journals in Education, which indexes over 700 publications. Includes information pertaining to health, physical education, and recreation, as well as all other fields of education. 1966–present.	National Institute of Education, Washington, DC and ERIC Processing and Reference Facility, Bethesda, MD	BRS SDC DIALOG
Excerpta Medica	Biomedical Sciences: One of the two principal sources for searching biomedical literature. Contains abstracts and citations of articles from 3500 biomedical journals published throughout the world, covering the entire field of human medicine and related disciplines. Online file corresponds to the 43 separate specialty abstract journals and 2 literature indexes which make up the printed Excerpta Medica, plus an additional 100,000 records annually that do not appear in the printed journals. Provides abstracts not only in all fields of medicine but also in drug and pharmaceutical literature and other health-related sciences. June 1974–present.	Excerpta Medica, Amsterdam, The Netherlands	AMANET SDC DIALOG
Foundation Directory	Descriptions of 3200 foundations with assets of $1 million or more which make grants of $100,000 or more annually. Useful when one is seeking sources of funding. Current year's data only.	Foundation Center, New York, NY	DIALOG

FSTA (Food Science and Technology Abstracts)	Food Science/Nutrition: Covers source documents related to all human food commodities, including world-wide patents, books, standards, and journal articles. Subject areas include basic food sciences, microbiology, hygiene, toxicology, specific food groups, legislation, etc. 1969–present.	International Food Information Service	SDC DIALOG
Grants	Source to more than 1500 grant programs available through government, commercial organizations, associations, and private foundations; academic disciplines for which grants are available are given with each program. Helpful when seeking funding for special projects. 1977–present.	Oryx Press, Phoenix, AZ	SDC DIALOG
Health Health-Tex	"Lay Persons" Physician's Desk Reference; health information.		Compu-Serve
Health Planning and Administration	Health economics, administration, and planning.	National Library of Medicine	BRS
International Pharmaceutical Abstracts	Provides information on all phases of the development and use of drugs and professional pharmaceutical practice. Scope ranges from the clinical, practical, and theoretical to the economic and scientific aspects; abstracts reporting clinical studies include study design, numbers of patients, dosage, dosage forms, and schedule. 1970–present.	American Society of Hospital Pharmacists, Washington, DC	DIALOG BRS
Life Sciences Collection	Contains abstracts of published information in fields of animal behavior, biochemistry, ecology, entomology, toxicology and virology, among others; covers books, journal articles, conference proceedings, and report literature. 1978–present.	Information Retrieval Ltd. London, England	DIALOG

(Continued)

Table 2.1. (Continued)

Database Name	Subject Area/Summary	Producer	Vendor
LIBCON LC/LINE	Extensive coverage of the monographic literature and nonprint materials cataloged by the Library of Congress; includes MARC records distributed by LC and MET records keyed by 3-M from LC depository cards.	SDC Search Service	SDC
MEDLARS/MEDLINE	Biomedical Sciences: Basically identical to MEDLINE (Medical Literature Analysis and Retrieval System). Contains references to citations from 3000 biomedical journals. Contains citations for current year plus two previous years; back files contain citations for earlier years to 1966. One of the two principal sources for searching biomedical literature.	National Library of Medicine, Bethesda, MD	BRS DIALOG
MEDOC	Government documents in the health sciences.	Eccles Health Sciences Library, University of Utah	BRS
Mental Health Abstracts	Worldwide information related to mental health. 1969–present.		DIALOG
Microcomputers Index	Subject/abstract guide to articles from over 21 microcomputer journals. 1980–present.	Microcomputer Information Services, Santa Clara, CA	DIALOG
National Foundations	Provides records of all 21,000 U.S. foundations which award grants, regardless of the assets of the foundation or the total amount of grants it awards annually. Includes 17,000 smaller foundations not listed in the Foundation Directory.	The Foundation Center, New York, NY	DIALOG

Name	Description	Provider	Service
National Newspaper Index	Indexes the Christian Science Monitor, New York Times, Wall Street Journal. Provides adjunct in such areas as food and nutrition and others.	Information Access Corporation, Los Altos, CA	DIALOG
Pharmaceutical News Index	Drug Literature: Indexes the drug industry's newsletters; ca. 1200 citations per month.	Data Counter, Inc. 620 South 5th St., Louisville, KY 40202	DIALOG
Psychological Abstracts/ PsychINFO	Psychology/Behavioral Sciences: Indexes and abstracts over 900 periodicals and 1500 books, technical reports, and monographs to provide coverage of original research, reviews, discussions, theory, conference reports, panel discussions, case studies, and descriptions of apparatus. 1967–present.	American Psychological Association, Washington, DC	DIALOG BRS SDC
PRE-MED	Current Clinical Medicine.	Bibliographic Retrieval Services, Inc.	BRS
RINGDOC	Covers 400 of world's scientific journals to provide extensive coverage of pharmaceutical literature. July 1964–present.	Derwent Publications Ltd.	SDC
SCISEARCH	Every Area of Pure and Applied Sciences: Multidisciplinary index to literature of science and technology prepared by the Institute for Scientific Information. Contains all records contained in printed Science Citation Index and Current Contents; includes 90% of the world's significant scientific and technical literature. January 1974–present.	Institute for Scientific Information, Philadelphia, PA	DIALOG

(Continued)

Table 2.1. (Continued)

Database Name	Subject Area/Summary	Producer	Vendor
SOCIAL SCISEARCH/ SSCI	Social Sciences Citation Index: Multidisciplinary data base indexing significant items from 1000 social sciences journals throughout the world as well as 2200 additional journals in the natural, physical, and biomedical sciences.	Institute for Scientific Information, Philadelphia, PA	DIALOG BRS
SPORT	Sports: Coverage of individual sports, practice, training, equipment, recreation, sports medicine, nutrition, injuries, treatment, sports facilities management and architecture, and international sports history. 1949–present.	Coaching Association of Canada's Sport Information/ Resource Centre, Ottawa, Ontario, Canada	SDC
SSIE (Smithsonian Science Information Exchange)	Contains reports of both government and privately funded research projects currently in progress or initiated and completed within the last 2 years.	Smithsonian Science Information Exchange, Washington, DC	DIALOG BRS SDC
WPI (World Patent Index)	Comprehensive and authoritative file containing documents relating to patent specifications issued by patent offices of major industrial nations.	Derwent Publications, Inc.	SDC

For extensive listing of databases available through a wide range of vendors consult *Omni Online Database Directory*, by M. Edelhart and O. Davies (New York: Macmillan, 1983).

supplement are particularly useful and can save the expense of printing retrospective citations online.

All documents for which citations are listed in SPORT and its print counterparts are owned by SIRC, and copies may be requested for a nominal charge ($2 per article, or 10¢ per page for articles over 30 pages). Individuals may order reprints directly from SIRC.

MEDLINE

The largest online database devoted to coverage of medicine and its allied fields is the MEDLINE (MEDLARS-on-line) database produced by the National Library of Medicine (NLM). MEDLINE, as of January 1982, contained citations to over 3,600,000 documents and was updated with over 20,000 citations monthly from some 3,000 journals published throughout the world. MEDLINE is currently available commercially through Bibliographic Retrieval Service (BRS) ($15 per hour plus telecommunications costs and royalties of $4 per connect hour) and Lockheed's DIALOG ($20 per hour plus telecommunications costs); authorized NLM-member medical libraries may also search MEDLINE directly through connect with NLM.

The printed counterparts to MEDLINE are the *Index Medicus* (and *Abridged Index Medicus*), *Index to Dental Literature*, and *International Nursing Index*, each of which is published monthly. A more concise printed tool for access to sports medicine information contained on MEDLINE, however, has been published by the President's Council on Physical Fitness and Sports since 1978. Entitled *Physical Fitness/Sports Medicine*, this quarterly index includes selected citations from MEDLINE. Primary access to information contained in this bibliography is by subject, but an author index is also included. (The online database can be searched through any combination of words contained in the entire citation.) The printed bibliography does not contain abstracts, but citations found online through MEDLINE often do.

Both the *Physical Fitness/Sports Medicine* bibliography and MEDLINE contain citations to a greater number of medicine and "pure science" publications than SPORT and its printed counterparts but do not include some of the important non-medical publications which SPORT includes. There is some overlap between the two, but this is not as much as might be expected—an informal survey of 220 publications received by the U.S. Olympic Committee's Sports Medicine Library shows that 87 are totally indexed through SPORT, 14 by MEDLINE, with only 6 being duplicately indexed by both.

This author has found that, in most cases, it is wise to search both MEDLINE and SPORT when comprehensive results are desired.

Documents indexed through MEDLINE are all available through the Regional Medical Library Network. Patrons must go through their library's interlibrary loan channels to request articles through this network. Documents may also be ordered online through Lockheed's DIALOG.

AMANET

The reader should refer to Table 2.1 for a listing of additional relevant databases. Which to search will, again, vary according to topic and depth of information desired.

One recent specialized database which has proven extremely useful is the American Medical Association's AMANET, which is distributed solely through the GTE Telenet Corporation. This contains current information related to drugs, procedures, and terminology, as well as the *Excerpta Medica* database (described in Table 2.1).

Printed Indexes

The sports medicine practitioner needs also to be aware of several important printed indexes which do not have online counterparts.

The *Physical Education Index*, published quarterly since 1978, is similar to the *Reader's Guide* in format. This index provides subject access to 170 English language journals relative to health, physical education, sports, recreation, and sports medicine, as well as to selected reports and biographies. A unique feature is its index to book reviews. This work, which is published by Ben Oak Publishing Company, is perhaps the second most comprehensive for sports medicine in general—in the previously mentioned survey of 220 publications received by the U.S. Olympic Committee Sports Medicine Library, 58 were indexed by the *Physical Education Index*, with 53 being duplicately indexed by SPORT and 7 also indexed by both MEDLINE and SPORT. There is no indication of the availability for ordering of publications listed in the *Physical Education Index*, so one would need to utilize one's local library and/or interlibrary loan channels to access cited documents.

Another significant printed index to which no online counterpart is available at present is the *Sport Documentation Monthly Bulletin* published by the Sports Documentation Centre of the University of

Birmingham, England. This work provides access to information contained in 109 journals from around the world and includes some non-English language publications not indexed elsewhere. Of the 220 USOC-received publications surveyed, this source indexed 43, with 30 duplicately indexed by SPORT, 11 by MEDLINE, and 25 by the *Physical Education Index*.

Role of the U.S. Olympic Committee

In 1981, the U.S. Olympic Committee began initial steps toward establishment of a comprehensive sports medicine database, with the hope of ultimately eliminating the need for cross-searching of so many databases when seeking sports medicine information. Initially, a sports medicine library/information center was established and an inhouse database created as an access tool to the USOC's own collection. By summer 1984, this database was an access tool to the USOC's own collection. By summer 1985, this database will be accessible to all users of the USOC's computer system at the Olympic Complex; ultimately, the database may be made available through dialup by remote users from around the country. Currently, the database contains records for some 3,500 books, periodicals, brochures and pamphlets, conference proceedings, reports, and article reprints, now owned by the USOC Sports Medicine Library, soon to be merged into the database are records for thousands of newspaper articles relevant to Olympic Sports published since 1980. At present, no effort is being made to index fully the materials received by the library, since staff is too small and funds limited; for now, existing online databases and printed indexes are utilized. Ultimately, plans are for the USOC to index fully its own collection, thereby creating the abovementioned comprehensive database; it has been proposed that the USOC enter into a cooperative agreement with SIRC/SPORT, whereby the USOC would coordinate documentation and indexing of relevant publications in the U.S., and the feasibility of such an arrangement is now being explored and a workshop scheduled for fall 1984 will gather selected experts and representatives from other sports/sports medicine organizations to discuss future potential cooperation for the mutual good of all. With this in mind, the USOC's initial (inhouse) database has been modeled closely after SPORT. Besides providing access to its own collection, the USOC provides access to the wealth of information available elsewhere through interlibrary loan services and through online literature search services using all existing vendors. The USOC will provide service to the public when time permits, but sometimes demand exceeds staff capability and response is slower than ideal.

Nonbibliographic Databases

This discussion has focused on retrieval of bibliographic information. Online access to nonbibliographic information within sports medicine (for example, training/competition statistics, medical data and injury records, etc.) presents special problems; the software to facilitate this type of retrieval on a mass scale is in its infancy, and many institutions which produce this kind of data prefer that it remain their confidential property.

FUTURE TRENDS

International cooperation, and cooperation between database producers, will likely become more and more important as information retrieval services proliferate, making possible more efficient translation and exchange of information.

The growing popularity of home and office computer systems will undoubtedly have an impact on the availability of access to sports medicine-related information, and more owners of home computers will likely "sign-on" for service from database vendors. It is likely that software will become more sophisticated, and perhaps at the same time more "user friendly," so that more and more individuals can utilize online databases.

CHAPTER 3

The United States Olympic Committee Drug Control Program

Kenneth S. Clarke

For years, the USOC, the ACSM, the American Medical Association (AMA), and other national organizations devoted to the health of athletes have disseminated current accurate information related to perceived drug use practices of athletes. Were it not for anabolic steriods, one would have confidence that these drug education programs were respected and reasonably effective. The deep belief among athletes, users or not, however, in both the advantage that these drugs give to athletes and the absence of visible evidence of their dangers have produced a tolerance at best among athletes for those who advance drug education positions. Worse, those who have perpetuated inaccurate information, regardless of motivation, have been given increasing credibility among these athletes. They have given responses to "How can I beat the system" and "How late can I quit steroids before drug testing" that the true experts could not give—because the substantiating data simply wasn't there.

At the 1983 Pan American Games in Caracas, things changed. For the first time, both technology and technicians were equal to the challenge of detecting use of anabolic steroids and testosterone. Drug testing not only caught users who had followed their experts' advice as to when to quit and/or how to mask such use, but it also

The Elite Athlete, edited by N. K. Butts, T. T. Gushiken, and B. Zarins. Copyright © 1985 by Spectrum Publications, Inc.

led to the American public's full support of a crackdown by the USOC even if the outcome might mean a few less medals. With this support and technology offered to the U.S. by the IOC-certified lab in Cologne until a U.S. lab could reach the same proficiency, the USOC Drug Control Program was created.

The USOC Drug Control Program is a drug-testing system that is equivalent to the International Olympic Committee's Doping Control Program and compliant with "human rights" and "chain of custody" expectations. Essentially, the USOC Drug Control Program is a service provided by the USOC to the sports' national governing bodies (NGBs) that enables urine collection at specific occasions and laboratory analysis for substances banned by the International Olympic Committee.

The USOC Drug Control Program can be requested by an NGB for *formal* or *informal* purposes. The *formal* option would lead to punitive action if an athlete is found to be positive for a banned substance. The *informal* option permitted by some organizations permits educational or research experiences to be applied. At the registration for any NGB event or team, the athlete is to be informed if formal drug testing is to be applied. Participation then will constitute informed athlete consent to be subject to the drug control process if selected. Subsequent noncompliance can be grounds for the same punitive action as being found positive for a banned substance. Policies as to the nature of the punitive action are the prerogative of the organization with jurisdiction.

Any physician, coach, athletic trainer, or other attendant of an athlete with a positive finding who is shown to have aided or abetted that offense is subject to at least the same action(s) as taken against that athlete.

Athlete Responsibilities

Selection of the athlete for testing will be determined by the occasion. At the Olympic Trials, every athlete selected to represent the U.S. will undergo formal testing; a positive finding for a banned substance will be cause for disqualification, and the athlete's replacement must likewise be tested. If Trials are conducted more than 60 days prior to the games, those athletes are subject to further formal testing closer to the games.

At other NGB-initiated occasions using formal testing, both medalists and nonmedalists will be subject to testing (e.g., top three and three others at random). At informal testing, the occasion is opportunity, not obligation, for experiencing the drug-testing process; the sponsoring organization will honor the confidentiality of the athlete's analysis results.

If selected for testing, the athlete will be notified of such personally by a USOC courier at the conclusion of his/her event and told to report to the Drug Control Station within 60 minutes. The courier will accompany the athlete until he/she so reports. The athlete then selects a code number and a beaker for urine collection. After providing the specimen under observation by a member of the USOC crew, he/she will select a sealed bag of two bottles, unseal the bag, and pour the specimen equally into the bottles. Each bottle then will be capped, crimped, sealed with wax, and coded in the presence of the athlete as his/her Specimen A and B.

Urine remaining in the beaker after the specimen bottles are sealed will be tested for pH; if alkaline, the athlete will be detained until strongly acid urine is provided. The athlete will sign that all these procedures were followed, and the crew chief will secure the bottles in a specially designed and identified shipping case.

Chain of Custody

The USOC will have a shipping agent pick up and sign for all cases from the Drug Control Station at the conclusion of the occasion and take them to the airplane at which time the airline will give a signature receipt. At the destination, another agent will give signature of receipt and take the cases directly to the laboratory where delivery of the cases will be accepted with the final signature of receipt. In each instance, "signature" attests that the seal on each shipping case is intact. Documentation of all signatures in the chain of custody is sent to USOC.

Laboratory Procedures

The USOC will select one or more laboratories that meet IOC standards for capability in detecting the categories of drugs on the IOC banned list. The laboratory first will analyze Specimen A of each coded pair. If Specimen A reveals the presence of a banned substance, the laboratory will recheck its findings with another sample from Specimen A. If confirmed, Specimen B for that code number will be analyzed after notifying the athlete as described below. The results of the analysis of Specimen B shall be final.

Chain of Communication

The USOC will provide the physician who is serving on site as its drug-testing crew chief with a range of codes from which the athletes at that occasion can select. The crew chief will maintain both the "Master Code" as it materializes and a "Manifest" of the codes of the bottles (i.e., no names) to be enclosed in a given shipping case. For formal drug testing occasions, the Master Code is sent to the chief executive officer of the organization with principal jurisdiction (USOC for Trials), with the crew chief keeping a confidential copy secured for backup. For informal testing occasions, the crew chief will keep the Master Code. The Manifest is placed inside the shipping case, and a copy is sent to USOC.

The laboratory results (Specimen A) will be phoned or telexed to USOC and confirmed subsequently by documentation. USOC will inform the person holding the Master Code of the respective findings by code number.

If the occasion is formal and the results are positive, the executive officer will contact the athlete by phone and overnight/signature-required letter that Specimen B will be analyzed within ten days of the contact between the executive officer and the athlete. Because of the decentralized nature of the program, the athlete may not be able to be present at the lab nor represented by a person of their selection, even though these options are offered. If this is the case, a surrogate athlete representative system would be employed to ensure that Specimen B is indeed of the right code number and remains free of evidence of tampering.

The result of Specimen B's analysis is final, and the principal organization's chief executive officer as well as the athlete is notified of it. The consequent action taken is the prerogative of the organization with jurisdiction in accordance with its existing policies. USOC then will prepare a confidential report of the aggregate data from all tested athletes for the USOC and associated NGB.

Appeal Process

Any athlete who is found to be positive for a banned substance has the right to register an appeal to the USOC Secretary-General. The USOC Secretary-General will implement appropriate procedures to review the appeal in a manner consistent with the USOC constitution and by-laws.

On Beating the System

The well-designed drug testing system theoretically can be beaten, perhaps, only by taking drugs that are not among or chemically related to those on the "Banned List." With the IOC List of Banned Drugs gaining in entries each quadrennium, the athlete who is resolved to resort to drugs for athletic purposes has few options within this "loophole." By "perhaps" is meant that each category of drugs on the IOC banned list includes the catch-all phrase, "and related compounds;" that which the athlete believes is not listed may indeed be cause for punitive action by being "related." By "theoretically" is meant that on a given day any system can suffer from a nonsystematic human or machine error. The athlete who counts on such, however, is playing Russian Roulette with five bullets in a six-cylinder revolver.

Many efforts to beat the system have been attempted. Some are quite imaginative.

1. At the drug control station, a trained member of the drug control crew will be assigned to the athlete for observing the athlete continuously, including the urination and the delivery of the container to the physician in charge. If the athlete cannot pass urine immediately, he/she will be provided liquid and patience; the athlete is detained until the specimen is given.

2. If a user-athlete had tried catheterization to empty his bladder and refill with the urine of someone else, it will not work. First, the kidney will continue to produce the athlete's urine and thereby will "contaminate" the surrogate urine with evidence of the banned substance. Further, a a person's urine is like a fingerprint. It is specifically peculiar to the individual in its nature, and the presence of two person's urine is detectable.

3. If the athlete had tried to "doctor" his/her own urine, it will not work. Sodium bicarbonate or other alkalizing agents may confuse drug analysis efforts, but the drug control program checks the pH of the urine specimen before the athlete leaves the station. If it is alkaline, the athlete is targeted for special attention, detained until his/her urine becomes strongly acid, and then noted for the most careful of attention at the lab.

4. If the athlete had taken a diuretic to dilute the urine, the laboratory will concentrate any dilute urine before beginning the analysis. *Any* urine that is "different" (including presence of a radioactive substance, multiple drugs, etc.) will be given special attention.

5. Until recently, most user-athletes tried to "beat the system" by stopping the use of a banned drug days or weeks before a competition. This no longer works for hormonal drugs: estimates for being clean after ceasing use are now in months, not weeks. Consequently, anyone who is truly confident that he/she stopped in time has lost by the time of competition whatever performance advantage they may have gained as a user (whether from psychological or physiological phenomena). Further, the body's clearance rate of hormonal drugs from the urine can look more like a roller-coaster than a ski jump. The vagaries of metabolism may show the athlete negative on one day and positive the next. Concentrating on one's training program only and not worrying about detection of past use is the nonuser's advantage.

Athletes and others in sport are encouraged to share anonymously or directly any question they may have and/or rumor of a new way that athletes from any country are attempting to mask the use of a banned substance so that all possibilities can receive attention. Contact the USOC Sports Medicine Division "Hotline," 1750 East Boulder Street, Colorado Springs, Colorado 80909 (1-800-233-0393).

II.
Biomechanics

CHAPTER **4**

Overview of the United States Olympic Committee Sports Medicine Biomechanics Program

Charles J. Dillman

Researchers in sports biomechanics are employing engineering principles and methodologies to solve three critical problems within the total realm of physical activity and sport. These problems are (1) determination of optimum *techniques* for performance in sports events, (2) investigation of *stresses* placed upon the body during the performance of activities; and (3) the design of sports *equipment*.

These three problems can be uniquely grouped because solutions to these questions require investigations into the mechanical aspects of human performance. Thus, through the studies of movements and forces that occur during the performance of a sports skill, investigators can obtain solutions to problems centered around technique, stress, and equipment requirements.

Recognizing the potential contribution that this field could make to amateur sports, the United States Olympic Committee (USOC) began in 1977 to develop a program of biomechanical services for amateur athletes. This initial effort was led by Dr. Gideon Ariel who developed a Biomechanics Laboratory at the Olympic Training Center in 1979. In the summer of 1981, due to increased demands

The Elite Athlete, edited by N. K. Butts, T. T. Gushiken, and B. Zarins. Copyright © 1985 by Spectrum Publications, Inc.

for services from this laboratory, the USOC expanded its commitment by hiring a full-time staff to conduct and coordinate biomechanical services requested by National Governing Bodies. The overall mission of the Sports Biomechanics Laboratory at the Olympic Complex is to conduct mechanical evaluations of various events and to make judgments as to how these factors are influencing the performance of our athletes who are in intensive training for international and Olympic competition.

SPECIFIC PROJECTS

The biomechanics program of the USOC is responsible for assisting 38 Olympic and Pan American sports. Since it is impossible for one laboratory to solve the many unique and varied problems for each of these sports, a national program of biomechanics has been established. The staff in Colorado Springs coordinates and supports the work of 23 biomechanists from throughout the U.S. to conduct studies for various national teams. Table 4.1 lists the projects and chief investigators who are presently participating in this program.

In order to provide an example of the results of several of these projects, the following reviews are presented of archery, cross-country skiing and ice hockey.

Archery: Evaluation of Stability and Release Factors

The purpose of this investigation is to determine the influence of three mechanical factors upon performance. The three biomechanical parameters of (1) body stability, (2) steadiness of sighting, and (3) arrow release have been analyzed for the 20 members of the National Team. Force platforms, the Selspot system, and high-speed films and video have been employed to investigate these factors.

Analysis of results has indicated that extreme levels of control and stability are needed for high performance. For example, sighting movements of one millimeter can result in a nine centimeters displacement of the arrow on the target. An oscillation of the body weight more than three millimeters during the release of the arrow can have a significant effect upon performance. Our results indicate that the best archers can control body and upper segment steadiness within these limits.

In addition, high-speed films have shown that the arrow actually "snakes" or oscillates in flight as it moves toward the target. This oscillation is caused by an angular torque placed upon the arrow at release. Minimizing this oscillation of the arrow would improve its flight toward the target and result in an improved performance. High-speed films and/or video of the finger release action have been used to aid the archer in minimizing the effect of this factor upon performance.

Cross-Country Skiing: A Comparison between Roller and On-Snow Skiing

A preliminary study was conducted to ascertain the technique differences between roller and snow skiing. Six skiers from the U.S. national team were filmed on the same day while performing roller and on-snow skiing. The athletes skied at various velocities under both conditions in an attempt to obtain a number of trials at similar speed. Standard biomechanical methods were used to analyze the performances. With respect to the limitations of this study (i.e., small sample of subjects, type of roller skis, amount of training on roller and snow skis prior to data collection, etc.), the following results appear warranted:

1. Significant differences do exist in the overall stride pattern between roller and on-snow skiing. When skiers are moving at approximately the same speed, the roller stride tends to be longer and at a slower frequency when compared with on-snow skiing.
2. The significant differences in stride characteristics between roller and snow skiing were primarily due to variations in the "kick phase" of the stride.
3. Analysis of leg segmental movement patterns performed during the kick indicated that there were significant differences between roller and snow skiing.

The findings of this initial investigation suggest that in attempts to make roller skiing more similar to snow skiing, athletes and coaches should focus upon the kick phase of the stride. It seems that if the kick on roller skis were performed quicker and from a more flexed position, especially at the knee joint, the two modes of skiing would become more similar in terms of the technical aspects of skiing.

Table 4.1.   USOC Biomechanical Sports Projects and Project Directors

Sport	Sports Projects	Directors
Archery	Evaluation of Stability and Release Factors in Archery	Charles J. Dillman, Ph.D., USOC, Department of Biomechanics and Computer Services
Bobsled	Starting Techniques in Bobsled	David A. Barlow, Ph.D., University of Delaware
Cross-Country Skiing	Comparison between Roller and On-Snow Skiing	Charles J. Dillman, Ph.D., USOC, Department of Biomechanics and Computer Services
Cycling	Pedaling Mechanics, Patho-mechanics, Aerodynamics and Movement Patterns of Elite Cyclists	Peter Cavanagh, Ph.D., The Pennsylvania State University; Peter Francis, Ph.D., San Diego State University; Robert C. Gregor, Ph.D., UCLA, and Chester Kyle, Ph.D., California State University at Long Beach
Decathlon	Technical Analysis of the Decathlon Events	Charles J. Dillman, Ph.D., USOC, Department of Biomechanics and Computer Services
Diving	Techniques of Elite Divers	Doris I. Miller, Ph.D., University of Washington
Fencing	Biomechanical Analysis of Elite Fencers	David A. Barlow, Ph.D., University of Delaware; Phillip J. Cheetham, USOC, Department of Biomechanics and Computer Services; Marius Valsamis, M.D., Brooklyn, New York; and PhDr. Aladar Kogler, CSc., Columbia University
Gymnastics	Preliminary Investigation of Various Gymnastics Techniques	Phillip J. Cheetham, USOC, Department of Biomechanics and Computer Services
Hammer Throw	Technique Analysis of Elite Hammer Throwers	Jesus Dapena, Ph.D., Indiana University
High Jumps	Technique Analysis of Elite High Jumpers	Jesus Dapena, Ph.D., Indiana University
Horizontal Jumps	Technique Analysis of the Horizontal Jumps in Athletics	James Hay, Ph.D., University of Iowa

(Continued)

Table 4.1. (Continued)

Sport	Sports Projects	Directors
Hurdles	Biomechanical Assessment of Elite Hurdlers	Ralph Mann, Ph.D., University of Kentucky, and Anne E. Atwater, Ph.D., University of Arizona
Ice Hockey	Speed Capabilities of Ice Hockey Players	Charles J. Dillman, Ph.D., USOC, Department of Biomechanics and Computer Services, and Nancy L. Greer, University of Massachusetts
Luge	Starting Technique in Luge	David A. Barlow, Ph.D., University of Delaware
Pole Vault	Technique Analysis of Elite Pole Vaulters	Peter McGinnis, University of Oregon
Race Walking	Technique and Force Platform Analysis of Race Walking	Charles J. Dillman, Ph.D., USOC, Department of Biomechanics and Computer Services, and Leonard B. Jansen, USOC, Department of Biomechanics and Computer Services
Rowing	Biomechanical Factors in Rowing	William Nelson, Crown Center Redevelopment Corp., Kansas City, Missouri
Shooting	Assessment of Stability in Shooting	Charles J. Dillman, Ph.D., USOC, Department of Biomechanics and Computer Services
Ski Jumping	Biomechanical Evaluations of the Take-Off Motion in Ski Jumping	Charles J. Dillman, Ph.D., USOC, Department of Biomechanics and Computer Services
Sprints	Technical Analysis of the Sprint and Hurdle Events	Ralph Mann, Ph.D., University of Kentucky, and Anne E. Atwater, Ph.D., University of Arizona
Swimming	Development of Propulsive Force by Swimmers	Ernie Maglischo, Ph.D., and Cheryl Maglischo, Ed.D., California State University at Chico
Synchronized Swimming	Techniques of Sculling Motions	Anne E. Atwater, Ph.D., University of Arizona, and Peter Francis, Ph.D., San Diego State University

(Continued)

Table 4.1.   (Continued)

Sport	Sports Projects	Directors
Table Tennis	Techniques of Forehand and Backhand Strokes	Jack Groppel, Ph.D., University of Illinois
Team Handball	Performance Analysis of the World's Top Teams	Kevin A. Campbell, Ph.D., University of Massachusetts
Throwing Events in Athletics	Biomechanical Analysis of the Throws in Athletics	Paul A. Ward, Ph.D., Holiday Spa; Robert C. Gregor, Ph.D., UCLA; Gideon B. Ariel, Ph.D., Coto Research Center
Volleyball (Men)	Individual Skills Analysis of Serve, Spike and Blocking	William A. Colvin, Ed.D., California State University at Chico, and Peter Francis, Ph.D., San Diego State University
Volleyball (Women)	Formation and Individual Skills Analysis of World's Best Teams	Gideon B. Ariel, Ph.D., Coto Research Center
Water Polo	Analysis of Throwing Technique	Robert C. Gregor, Ph.D., UCLA
Weightlifting	Analysis of Deviations in Center of Pressure and Bar Movements During Lifting	John J. Garhammer, Ph.D., International Maxachievement Institute

The frictional advantages of roller skis during the free glide phase and gliding while poling phase would seem to have a beneficial effect on the technique training for American skiers. Our previous research indicates that the U.S. skiers need to obtain a greater feeling for free gliding and continuation of gliding while poling. Roller skis would seem to facilitate the acquisition of these skills which are needed to ski faster at the world level of competition.

Ice Hockey: Speed Capabilities of Ice Hockey Players

The purpose of this project was to conduct an assessment of the speed capabilities of top amateur hockey players. In order to investigate the quickness of ice hockey players, two and three dimensional high-speed films were taken during games and while performing reaction-speed and acceleration tests.

Analysis of movement and velocity patterns of ice hockey players during games indicated that they frequently react to various situations with short periods of accelerations lasting only between one and two seconds. In order to evaluate these specific speed requirements, a reaction speed test has been developed. Preliminary analysis of performance on this test indicates that the velocity patterns observed during a game are closely simulated in our reaction-speed protocol.

Based upon a biomechanical analysis of an acceleration test performed from a stationary start, we have determined that the speed of American players could be significantly improved if leg forces were applied from a more flexed position. This adjustment would result in a greater proportion of the available force being applied in the desired direction of motion. If this change in technique could be made, we have estimated that a player could increase his range of movement by three feet during an initial two-second period of acceleration.

SUMMARY

As part of the total Olympic Sports Medicine Program, the USOC has made a significant commitment to the area of biomechanics. Over the last several years, a national program of biomechanical assistance has been developed to solve critical performance problems for selected national teams. There is no doubt that researchers in biomechanics are making a significant contribution to the development of amateur athletes within the Olympic program.

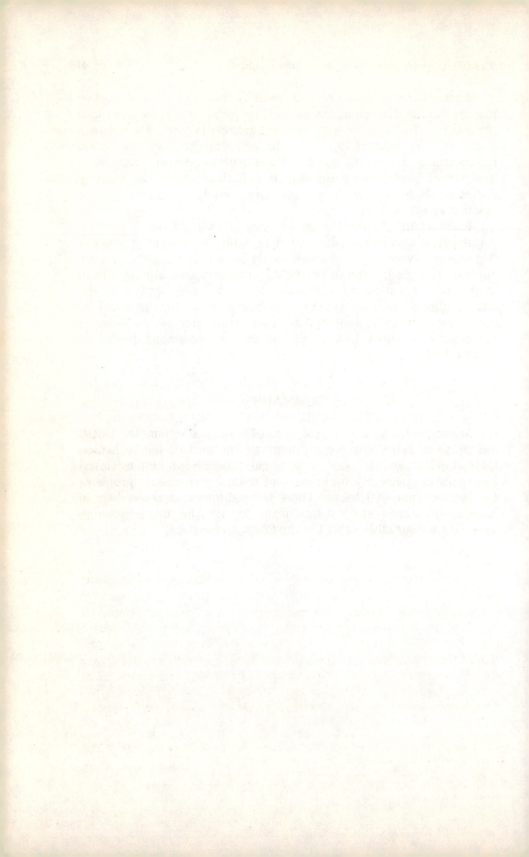

CHAPTER **5**

Biomechanical Analysis of the Elite Sprinter and Hurdler

Ralph Mann

As indicated in earlier chapters, in 1982 the United States Olympic Committee (USOC) began funding the Elite Athlete Project in an effort to utilize the area of sport science to better prepare the Olympic-caliber athlete. The program was initiated, to a large extent, due to the existence of similar programs that have been an established part of the Olympic development program of a number of Eastern-bloc countries. The success of these programs indicated that the U.S. athlete was not being provided sufficient feedback to best develop his/her available talent. To remedy this problem, experts in medicine, exercise physiology, sports psychology, and biomechanics were recruited to provide relevant feedback in each of their respective areas.

The Athletics Congress (TAC) was one of the National Governing Bodies (NGB) that was funded under the Elite Athlete Project. In the sprint and hurdle events, it was decided that a major effort was to be directed toward biomechanically analyzing men and women athletes. The primary goal of this effort was to identify the mechanical weaknesses of the involved athletes and to get the results to the coaches so that the problems could be remediated. The secondary goal was to build a database in an effort to quantify the parameters inherent in a successful sprint or hurdle performance.

The Elite Athlete, edited by N. K. Butts, T. T. Gushiken, and B. Zarins. Copyright © 1985 by Spectrum Publications, Inc.

As recipient of the grant for biomechanical analysis, the laboratory staff at the University of Kentucky decided to divide the project into two phases: (1) kinematic-based investigation focused on actual competitive situations, and (2) kinetic-based investigations in controlled, noncompetitive situations. The kinematic information was to be application-oriented to each individual and delivered to the athlete's coach within two weeks of the competition from which it was collected. The kinetic information was to be application-oriented to both the group and the individual and was scheduled to be collected toward the end of the year so that specific problems could be studied in a controlled situation. This information was to be delivered at the conclusion of the competitive year, with emphasis on improvement for the next competitive season.

For each area of performance (sprints or hurdles), and each type of analysis emphasis (kinematic or kinetic), specific results were selected to identify the strengths and weaknesses of both the individual athlete and the group as a whole. The majority of the results reported were selected due to the relationship of the result to performance, as determined from previous research conducted on sprinting and hurdling [1-5]. A number of additional results were included on the request of the involved coaches, as the current research indicated a superior method of reporting a significant trend [6]. The following information indicates the current results of the data gathered to date.

THE SPRINTS: KINEMATIC RESULTS

To rate the kinematic performance of a sprinter, it is necessary to identify certain total system as well as individual segment results. Results such as stride rate or stride length indicate how the total system is integrating the contributions of the segments toward performance. Individual results such as upper-leg orientation at specific positions or lower-leg rotational speed during selected phases denote how the body parts are contributing to performance. The examples presented in this section are for the elite athlete male 100-meter performers examined to date; however, except where indicated, the trends can be expanded to cover all short (100–200 meter) sprinters.

Stride Rate and Stride Length (Total Body Result)

The speed at which a sprinter moves his legs (stride rate) and how far each stride covers (stride length) determines the success of the performance. An ideal situation includes a high stride rate coupled

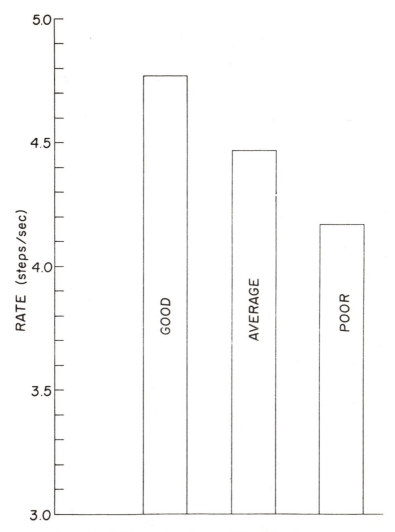

Figure 5.1. Stride rate for male elite athlete 100-meter sprinters.

with a large stride length. Figures 5.1 and 5.2 show the average stride rate and stride length for elite male 100-meter athletes. In addition, values indicating magnitude and direction of results deemed good and poor are indicated. In both figures, results shifted toward the poor category indicate a weakness in the sprint performance, while results shifted toward the good category can be beneficial if the corresponding value is not decreased. Thus, a high stride rate is good,

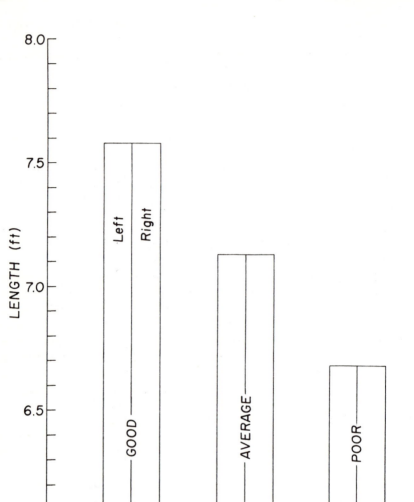

Figure 5.2. Stride length for male elite athlete 100-meter sprinters.

but only if stride length is maintained at an acceptable level. Likewise, a large stride length is beneficial, but only if an acceptable stride rate is maintained.

The most recent research on sprinting indicates that, in the short sprints, improvement in stride rate and length is done primarily during ground contact. Moreover, it appears that improvement in stride rate is the means by which the better sprinters improve their performance. Thus, the superior sprinter will maintain an acceptable or slightly above average stride length, while producing an excellent stride rate. Both results are improved by increasing leg strength so that the necessary ground forces can be produced more quickly, and improving running mechanics so that less energy is wasted while on the ground. The segmental results that follow identify how the elite sprinter maximizes stride rate through minimizing the ground contact time.

One final factor can affect stride rate and length results. If a performer is unusually tall or short, the results may be misleading. If leg length is taken into account, however, the stride/rate length ratio becomes comparable.

Total Body Vertical Speed (Total Body Result)

Although the performer must project the body vertically (upward) during the sprint, excessive vertical motion is not wanted. Figure 5.3 shows good, average, and poor levels of vertical speed for the elite male 100-meter athletes. The better sprinters tend to produce just enough vertical speed to allow time to complete leg recovery and prepare for the next ground contact, while directing more effort toward maintaining horizontal speed.

Lower-Arm Motion (Individual Segment Result)

Contrary to popular belief, the forearm (lower arm) does not maintain the same angle with the upper arm during sprinting. The angle normally ranges from a minimum at full front or full back position, to a maximum at the midpoint of the arm swing during each stride. Figure 5.4 indicates the average lower-arm motion for the elite male 100-meter sprinters. In addition, results indicating the performance levels deemed good and poor are also indicated. As indicated in Figure 5.4, average, or even insufficient, arm action is not a problem. Excessive arm action, however, signals that the sprinter is producing uneconomical motion, as well as overstriding.

Upper-Arm Motion (Individual Segment Result)

The motion of the upper arm can tell much about the quality of a sprinter. The upper arm normally comes in front of the body to

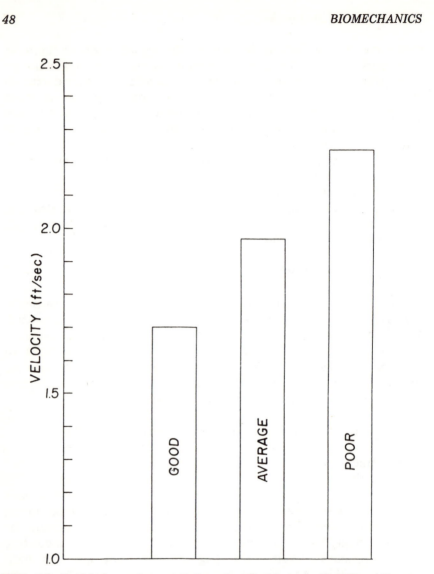

Figure 5.3. Total body maximum vertical speed attained by male elite athlete 100-meter sprinters.

about 45 degrees in relation to the trunk, then rotates to a maximum position in back of the body of about 80 degrees during each stride. Figure 5.5 indicates the typical upper-arm motion for the male 100-meter sprinters. For comparison, the performance shifts indicating beneficial or unwanted range of motion are also indicated. As in

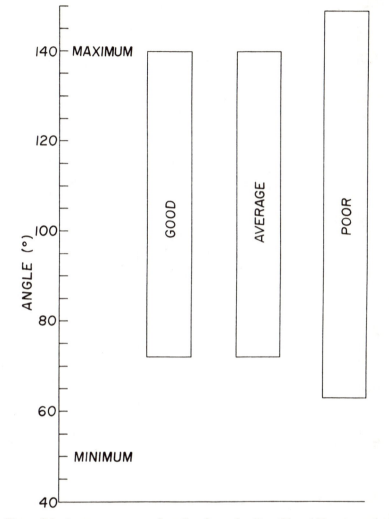

Figure 5.4. Lower-arm range of motion for male elite athlete 100-meter sprinters. The result identified is the angle formed between the arm (upper arm) and forearm (lower arm), with 180 degrees indicating full extension.

the lower-arm motion, insufficient arm action is usually not a problem, but excessive arm action indicates that the sprinter is producing uneconomical motion and denotes overstriding in the performance.

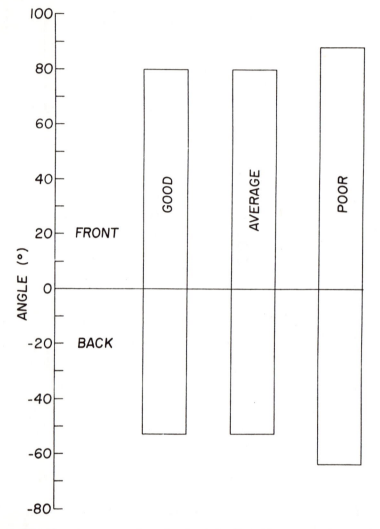

Figure 5.5. Upper-arm range of motion for male elite athlete 100-meter sprinters. The result identified is the angle formed between the trunk and arm (upper arm). Positive results indicate the upper arm is in front of the body, negative results indicate the upper arm is behind the body; zero identifies the point when the upper arm is aligned with the trunk.

Horizontal Foot Speed at Touchdown (Individual Segment Result)

When the foot contacts the ground in sprinting, it is moving forward (horizontally) with respect to the ground, resulting in a braking action which slows the sprinter. It has been found that the

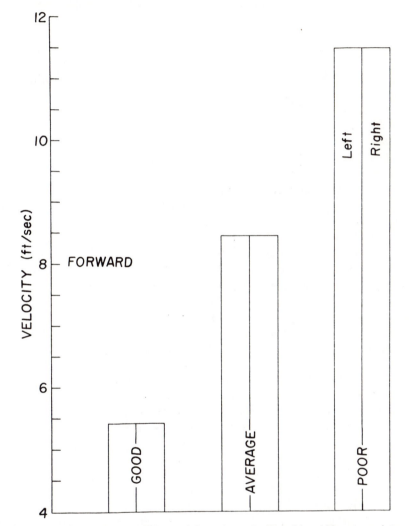

Figure 5.6. Horizontal foot speed at touchdown for male elite athlete 100-meter sprinters.

better sprinters recover the foot so that it is not moving forward as quickly as touchdown, effectively decreasing the braking force. Figure 5.6 shows the good, average, and poor forward foot speed results at touchdown for the elite male 100-meter sprinters. Although no sprinter has been able to recover the foot so that it is moving backward when it hits the ground, this should be the goal of every performer.

Horizontal Foot Distance from the Body at Touchdown
(Individual Segment Result)

To sprint properly, the foot must touch down in front of the body. This is a very important action since it increases stride length, as well as giving the leg a greater range of motion to produce the necessary vertical speed and maintain the forward motion while on the ground. On the other hand, the farther out the sprinter lands, and the greater the range of motion of the ground leg, the longer the ground time. Thus, a tradeoff situation occurs since sufficient leg range of motion is needed to produce the necessary ground forces and produce an acceptable stride length, while the ground time must be reduced to a minimum to maximize stride rate.

The most recent research on sprinting indicates that the better elite athlete sprinters are favoring a decrease in ground time over an increase in leg range of motion. Thus, they are actually minimizing the horizontal touchdown distance in an effort to minimize the ground time and maximize stride rate. This surprising result raises a number of questions concerning how the better sprinters are minimizing this touchdown distance. As shown by the stride length results (Figure 5.2), they are not sacrificing stride length in an effort to minimize ground time. From the available data, it is evident that the sprinters are minimizing ground time in two ways:

1. Properly preparing the ground leg for touchdown. (This is discussed in the section on leg motion and speed results.)
2. Developing sufficient leg strength to generate the necessary velocity changes during a shorter ground time. It must be realized that the biggest problem in sprinting is to stop the downward fall of the body and produce upward projection into the next airphase. To accomplish this, large vertical forces must be produced during ground contact. This combination of force and time, which is termed "impulse," amounts to about 50 ft•s for both average and elite sprinters. The difference is that the average sprinter exerts 400 pounds of force for .125 seconds of ground contact (400 X .125 = 50), while the elite sprinter exerts 500 pounds of force for .10 seconds of ground contact (500 X .10 = 50). Thus, the elite sprinters decrease ground time (which increases stride rate) without affecting the other performance results (like stride length) by having greater leg strength.

To minimize the touchdown distance, and get the most out of this action, the sprinter must be very strong in the hamstring and gluteal

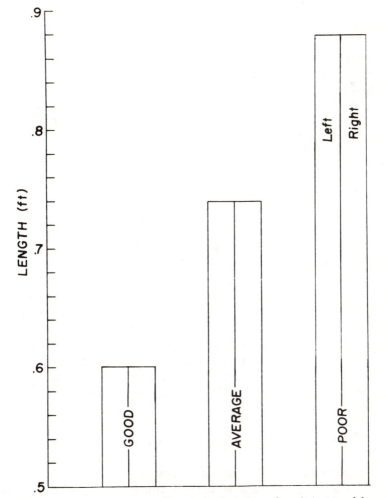

Figure 5.7. Horizontal foot distance from the body (center of gravity) at touchdown for male elite athlete 100-meter sprinters.

muscles since these are needed to pull the body over the touchdown point during the initial portion of ground contact. More than any other factor, the strength of these muscles dictate the success of a sprinter.

Figure 5.7 shows the average horizontal distance the foot is in front of the body at touchdown. In addition, those results constituting good and poor performance values are indicated. It must be remembered that touchdown distance is a tradeoff between the need to decrease ground time (to increase stride rate) and the need to produce the necessary ground forces (to maintain stride length). Thus, a small touchdown distance is good, as long as the rest of the sprint stride does not suffer. A good indicator of whether or not a performer can handle the touchdown distance is the stride length result (Figure 5.2). If the stride length is at least average, then the touchdown distance is acceptable. If the touchdown distance is large, then either the sprinter does not have sufficient leg strength, or is not preparing properly for ground contact.

Upper-Leg Angular Motion (Individual Segment Result)

There are three critical positions for the upper leg during sprinting: (1) the position at takeoff, (2) the full extension position, and (3) the full flexion position. Figure 5.8 shows good, average, and poor upper leg results for the elite male 100-meter sprinters. The better sprinters tend to minimize upper leg extension at takeoff (larger angle) and full extension (larger angle), and maximize upper leg flexion at full flexion (larger angle). These leg motions are produced to minimize ground time and make leg recovery as efficient as possible. It must be emphasized, however, that a very good angle at one position is only beneficial if the other results are acceptable. Poor results here commonly indicate a lack of leg strength (indicated by excessive extension at takeoff), or an inability of a performer to properly recover the leg (indicated by insufficient flexion at full flexion).

Upper-Leg Rotational Speed (Individual Segment Result)

Upper-leg rotational speed is critical in recovering the leg after takeoff (flexion), rotating it toward touchdown (extension), and finally, continuing the extension rotation during ground contact. Figure 5.9 shows good, average, and poor results for the maximum flexion speed of the upper leg during recovery, the extension speed at touchdown, and the average extension speed during the ground phase. The better sprinters tend to maximize the leg recovery and touchdown rotation speeds, while maintaining or actually increasing (larger than touchdown) leg speed during ground contact. As in upper-leg position (Figure 5.8), these values are directly related to the quality of the upper-leg strength, as well as sprinting mechanics.

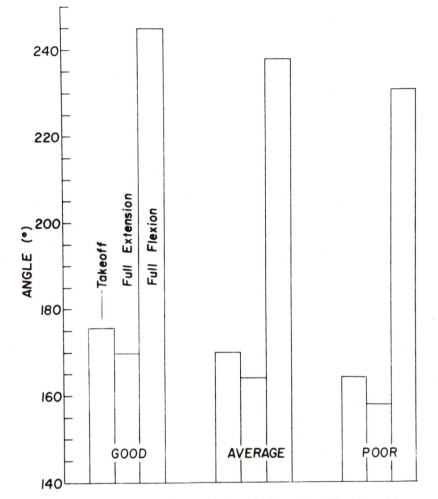

Figure 5.8. Thigh (upper leg) angular motion for male elite athlete 100-meter sprinters.

Lower-Leg Angular Motion (Individual Segment Result)

There are three critical positions for the lower leg during sprinting: (1) the position at takeoff, (2) the maximum flexion during recovery and (3) the position when the ankle crosses the opposite leg during recovery. Figure 5.10 shows good, average, and poor results for takeoff, maximum flexion, and the point where the ankle crosses

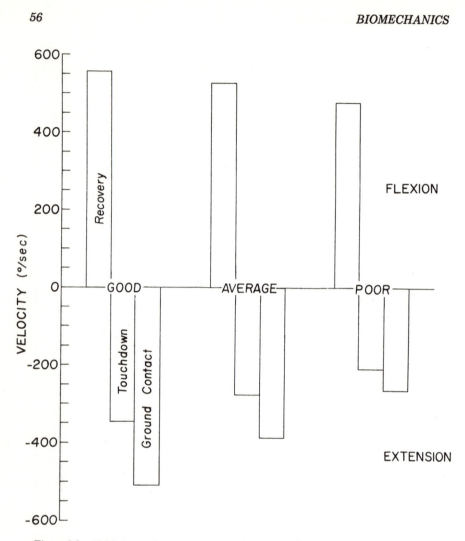

Figure 5.9. Thigh (upper leg) rotational speed for male elite athlete 100-meter sprinters.

the opposite leg. The better sprinters tend to minimize lower leg extension at takeoff (smaller angle) to minimize the ground contact time (to increase stride rate). Likewise, the superior performer minimizes the lower leg angle during both recovery (smaller angle) and as the ankle passes the opposite leg (smaller angle) to make the task of recovering the leg both faster and easier. Poor results here, as in the upper leg (Figure 5.8) commonly point to a lack of leg strength (indicated by excessive extension at takeoff), or an inability to properly recover the leg (indicated by insufficient flexion during recovery).

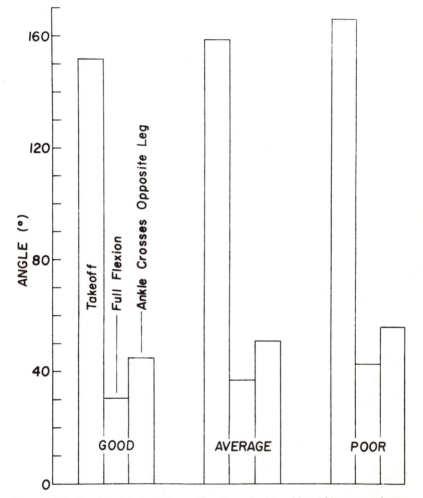

Figure 5.10. Leg (lower leg) angular motion for male elite athlete 100-meter sprinters.

Lower-Leg Rotational Speed (Individual Segment Result)

Lower-leg rotational speed is critical as touchdown occurs since it indicates the amount of braking (slowing down) that occurs during ground contact. The result for good, average, and poor rotational speeds of the lower leg at touchdown for the elite sprinters are presented in Figure 5.11. The better sprinters are able to complete

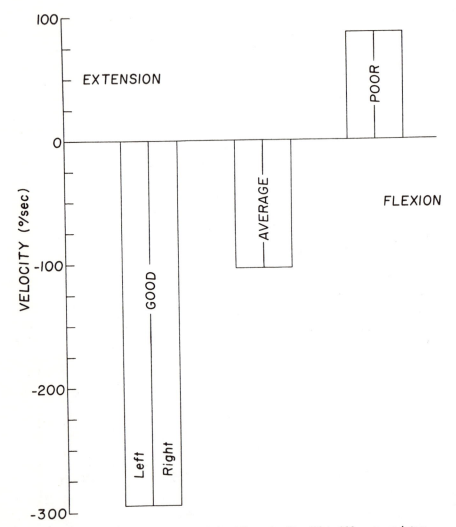

Figure 5.11. Leg (lower leg) rotational speed for male elite athlete 100-meter sprinters.

lower-leg extension in sufficient time during the air phase to be able to produce a significant amount of lower-leg flexion speed at touch-down. This results in a reduction in the forward braking force during the initial portion of ground contact.

THE SPRINTS: KINETIC RESULTS

From the kinematic results, it is evident that the action of the upper and lower legs are the keys to successful sprinting. It is also evident that strength is related to the performer's ability to produce the proper leg motions. The best direct measures of the leg strength and quality of the mechanics of a sprinter are the forces produced during ground contact. The vertical force indicates the effort expended to stop the fall of the body and project it upward, into the next air phase. The horizontal force directly measures the amount of unwanted braking during the initial portion of ground contact, as well as the amount of force needed to recover the lost forward speed. The following examples are for the elite athlete female 100-, 200-, and 400-meter sprinters examined to date; however, except where indicated, the trends can be expanded to apply to all sprinters.

Vertical Force

Although sprinting appears to be a horizontal (forward) movement, the majority of the effort expended once top speed has been attained is in the vertical (upward) direction. Since the sprint is a series of jumps, when a sprinter lands, the body is falling downward. This downward motion must be halted, and upward motion produced to project the body into the next stride. To halt this downward motion and produce upward movement, a large vertical force must be exerted by the sprinter while on the ground. Figure 5.12 shows the vertical ground forces produced by all of the elite athlete women sprinters tested to date. For comparison, values for good, average, and poor force production are identified. As indicated by Figure 5.12, since the average vertical ground force is about 320 pounds, and since a sprinter must produce this force about 30 times during a 100-meter race, it is evident that vertical force is a major contributor to fatigue. Additionally, since the force must be produced over a very small time period (about .11 second), it stresses the body to an even greater extent. The better sprinters, therefore, produce only sufficient vertical forces to ensure that the air phase is long enough to complete the leg recovery.

There are three productive ways to minimize the effects of the vertical force effort. The first is to develop great leg strength in the performer so that the demands of the force are less fatiguing. Second, proper sprint mechanics can avoid inefficient force production. Finally, the weight of the performer should be minimized by

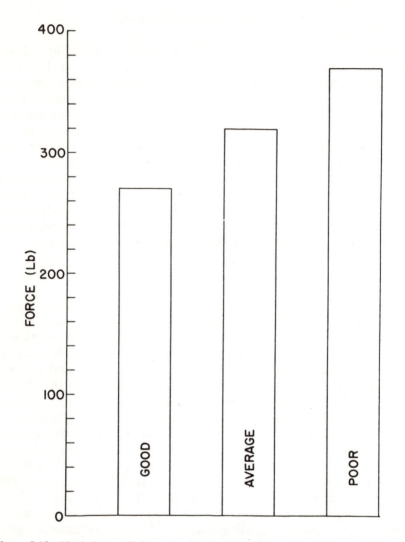

Figure 5.12. Vertical ground force for female elite athlete 100-, 200-, and 400-meter sprinters.

limiting all possible useless body fat and bulk that a sprinter must carry.

Horizontal Force

Since a sprinter only wants to maintain maximum horizontal velocity once it has been reached, there is little need to produce any horizontal (forward and backward) force while on the ground. Unfortunately, to place the legs in a position to produce the necessary vertical force (Figure 5.12), unwanted horizontal force is produced, which slows the body down during the first part of the ground phase. To maintain maximum horizontal velocity, therefore, the sprinter must produce a horizontal force, in the opposite direction, to speed up during the last portion of the ground phase. Figure 5.13 shows this pattern of negative (unwanted) force followed by positive (needed) force for all elite athlete women sprinters recorded to date. For both the negative and positive forces, values for good, average, and poor results are identified. As the figure indicates, the average horizontal forces in both directions are small compared to the vertical ground force. Since the negative horizontal force is unwanted and produced only because vertical force is needed, this force should be minimized. This can be done, without sacrificing the production of the needed vertical force, by using the hamstring and gluteal groups to pull the body over the touchdown leg during the first 20 to 30 percent of ground contact. This action demands great strength from a sprinter and is the cause of the majority of injuries sustained in sprinting. It is, however, the only way to economically produce the needed vertical force without hindering speed. This is evident since an equal positive horizontal force (integrated over time) is needed to offset the negative force; thus the negative force is minimized, and the amount of positive force needed to balance the negative force can be smaller. Figure 5.13 demonstrates this conclusion since those sprinters that produced small negative force only had to produce a small positive force to balance the effort. Likewise, those sprinters that produced a large negative force had to produce a large positive force.

If a sprinter does not possess great leg strength, there is another way to produce the needed vertical force. This is done by jamming the leg into the ground at touchdown. In this manner, the leg acts like a pole-vault pole and vaults the performer into the air. Unfortunately, this produces very high horizontal braking forces, which must be countered by very large positive forces during the second half of ground contact. This is, obviously, very energy wasteful and would severely reduce the endurance of the performance.

If a sprinter wants to decrease the horizontal braking force, yet does not have the strength to do so economically, it can be performed in another manner. The horizontal force can be decreased by simply eliminating the potential to use the leg as a vaulting pole. By placing the leg under (instead of in front of) the body at touchdown, the leg cannot be used to produce the unwanted braking force.

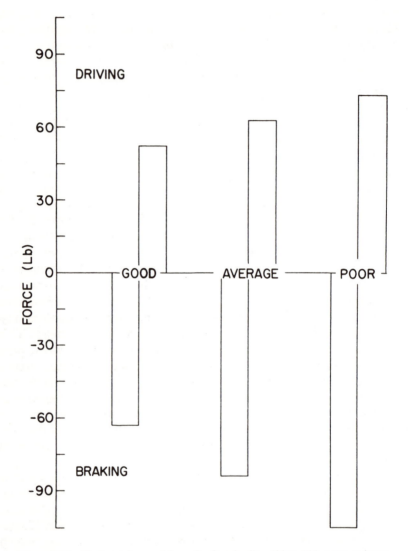

Figure 5.13. Horizontal ground force for female elite athlete 100-meter sprinters.

Unfortunately, it also cannot be used to produce the needed vertical force during the initial portion of ground contact. This would, of course, severely reduce the stride length of the performer, as well as reduce the time needed for the legs to recovery and prepare for the next ground phase.

It is evident that the only way to directly maximize the needed vertical force, while minimizing the unwanted braking force, is to utilize proper running mechanics, as well as to develop and use large muscle forces in the legs. Indirectly, the weight of the performer can be minimized, by ensuring that body fat, as well as all unnecessary upper-body bulk, is limited.

THE HURDLES: KINEMATIC RESULTS

As in sprinting, to rate the kinematic performance of a hurdler, it is necessary to identify both total system as well as individual segment results. The examples presented in this section are for the elite athlete male 110-meter hurdlers; however, except where noted, the trends can be expanded to apply to all hurdlers.

Stride Times between and over the Hurdles (Total Body Result)

Unlike sprint running, a number of the strides involved in the hurdle race are dissimilar. The first stride off of the hurdle should be short since the performer wants to get back on the ground as soon as possible. After this point, the stride should revert to a typical sprint stride until the stride prior to hurdle clearance (in the long hurdles this constitutes a number of strides; however, in the short hurdles the second stride is the only stride that is a typical sprint stride). The stride prior to hurdle clearance must be directed forward (not up) to prepare for the hurdle stride (much like a long jumper settles in the last strides prior to takeoff). Finally, the hurdle stride is altered to the greatest extent since the body must be projected vertically into the air more than normal. Figure 5.14 indicates good, average, and poor temporal results for each of the four strides for all male athlete elite short hurdlers analyzed to date. In addition, the total times are divided into ground and air times. For long hurdlers, the second stride time should be perpetuated until the stride prior to hurdle clearance.

Length of Hurdle Stride (Total Body Result)

Because of the need to elevate the body over the hurdle, the hurdle stride is longer than a normal stride. The amount of additional vertical motion should, however, be kept at a minimum. An excellent result indicating how efficiently a hurdle is negotiated is the length

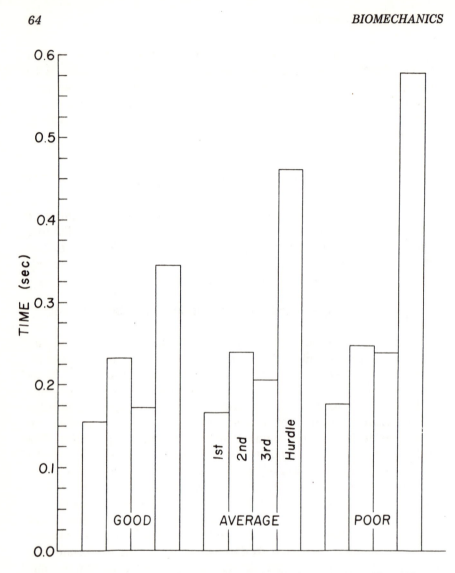

Figure 5.14. Stride times between and over the hurdle for male elite athlete 110-meter hurdlers.

of the hurdle stride and how it is divided. The shorter the stride, the more economical the motion since increased air time can only slow the performance. In addition, the distance from the body at the takeoff point to the hurdle should be greater than the distance from the hurdle to the body at the touchdown point to the performer to reach the highest point prior to the hurdle and be on the way down

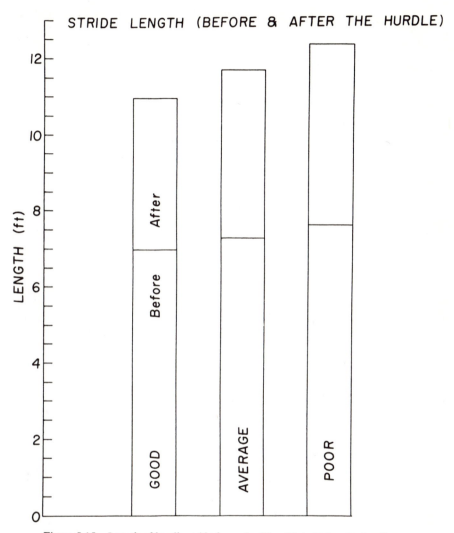

Figure 5.15. Length of hurdle stride for male elite athlete 110-meter hurdlers.

as the hurdle is cleared. This is necessary to properly clear the lead leg and allow it to regain ground contact without having to hesitate while the rest of the body comes off the hurdle. Figure 5.15 shows good, average, and poor results for the length of the hurdle stride, as well as how the stride is divided (before and after), for all elite athlete male short hurdlers analyzed to date.

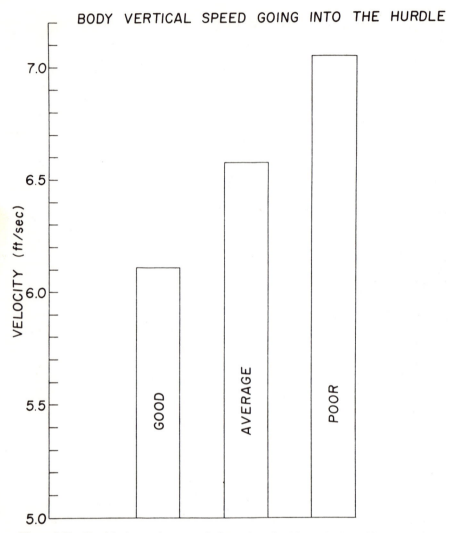

Figure 5.16. Total body maximum vertical speed attained by male elite athlete 110-meter hurdlers.

Body Vertical Speed Going into the Hurdle (Total Body Result)

The best measure of efficient hurdle technique can be found in the vertical (upward) speed of the body as it is projected over the hurdle. Figure 5.16 shows the good, average, and poor result for all male elite 100-hurdlers analyzed to date. The lower the vertical speed, the less time spent in the air, and the sooner the performer can regain ground contact and continue toward the next barrier. It is obvious, therefore, that this value should be minimized as much as possible.

Horizontal Foot Speed Going into and Coming off of the Hurdle (Individual Segment Result)

The hurdle stride demands some unique adaptations to the normal sprint stride in order to clear the barrier. Since the body must be projected higher into the air than normal, a large amount of vertical speed must be created during ground contact going into the hurdle. One of the ways vertical speed can be produced is to have the touchdown foot moving forward when ground contact occurs. Thus, when the ground stops the forward motion, it rotates the hurdler up and over the ground leg (similar to a pole vaulter using a steel pole). Another useful result from this action is that it produces forward rotation, which helps the hurdler move into the hurdle. Unfortunately, there is one major drawback to this action. The ground force that stops the foot (and produces the vertical speed) also slows down the forward speed of the hurdler. Although this method of producing vertical speed must be used to produce sufficient vertical lift, it should be minimized by either reducing the amount of vertical speed needed or produce it by other means. Better hurdlers tend to keep foot speed at touchdown low going into the hurdle and employ muscular strength (upper-leg extensors) to share in the production of vertical speed.

Coming off of the hurdle, the body should be directed forward again, since the strides between the hurdles are essentially sprint strides. Since a large amount of vertical speed is not needed until the next hurdle, foot speed at touchdown should be minimized to reduce the forward braking mentioned earlier. In fact, good hurdlers can actually have the foot moving backward as touchdown occurs after the hurdle. This eliminates virtually all forward braking and quickly moves the performer toward the next hurdle.

Figure 5.17 presents the foot speed results, both going into and coming off of the hurdle, for all male elite short hurdlers investigated to date. For comparison purposes, values for good, average, and poor results are indicated.

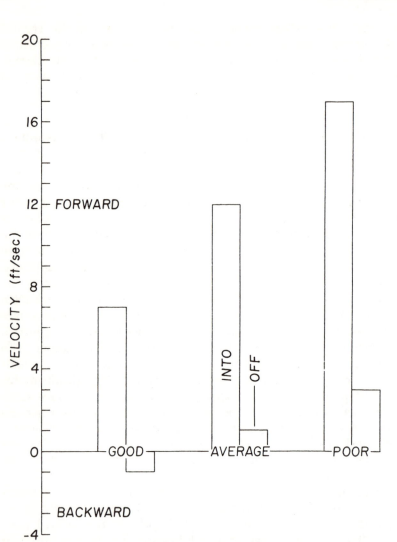

Figure 5.17. Horizontal foot speed at touchdown, going into and coming off of the hurdle, for male elite athlete 110-meter hurdlers.

Horizontal Foot Distance from the Body at Touchdown Going into and Coming off of the Hurdle (Individual Segment Result)

To properly negotiate the hurdle, the foot must touch down in front of the body going into the hurdle. This action is necessary to produce the vertical projection needed to clear the barrier, as well as giving the leg a greater range of motion to maintain the forward motion while on the ground. On the other hand, the farther out the hurdler lands, the greater the horizontal braking and the longer the ground time. Thus, a tradeoff situation occurs since sufficient range of motion is needed to produce the ground forces required for hurdle clearance, while the ground time must be reduced to a minimum to decrease forward braking and hurdle time.

The most recent research indicates that the better elite athlete hurdlers are favoring a decrease in ground time over an increase in leg range of motion. Thus, they are actually minimizing the horizontal touchdown distance in an effort to minimize ground time and horizontal braking. As in sprinting, the hurdlers are accomplishing this goal, while still producing proper hurdle clearance, in two ways:

1. Properly preparing the ground leg for touchdown going into the hurdle (this is discussed in the section on leg speed results).
2. Developing sufficient leg strength to generate the necessary velocity changes during a shorter ground time (as discussed in the sprint results on touchdown distance, and is further expanded in the hurdle kinetic results).

As in sprinting, the strength of the hamstring and gluteal muscles will dictate how close the hurdler can touch down in front of the body.

Coming off of the hurdle, since vertical speed is not critical, touchdown should occur directly under the body. In fact, good hurdlers land with the body directly over, or even ahead of, the touchdown point.

Figure 5.18 presents the foot distances, both going into and coming off of the hurdle, for the male elite athlete 110 hurdlers. For comparison, good, average, and poor values for all such athletes investigated to date are indicated.

Upper- and Lower-Leg Rotational Speed Going into the Hurdle (Individual Segment Result)

To get the most out of the legs during ground contact going into the hurdle, the upper and lower legs must possess great speed and strength. At touchdown, the upper leg should be extending slightly; then during ground contact, the speed of extension should be maximized. By extending at touchdown, the forward foot speed is reduced, which decreases the forward braking going into the hurdle

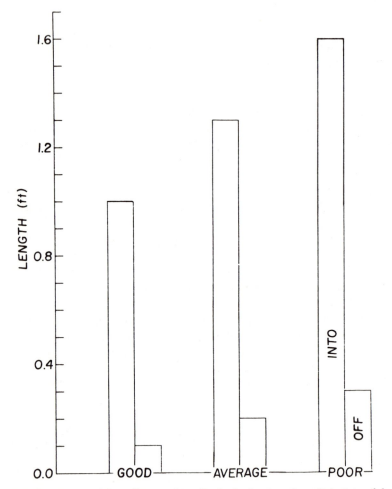

Figure 5.18. Horizontal foot distance from the body (center of gravity) at touchdown, going into and coming off of the hurdle, for male elite athlete 110-meter hurdlers.

(Figure 5.17). Then during ground contact, the increased speed of extension serves to project the hurdler toward the barrier.

The role of the lower leg during the stride going into the hurdle is to produce flexion going into the initial portion of ground contact, then quickly extend during the latter stages of contact. By flexing

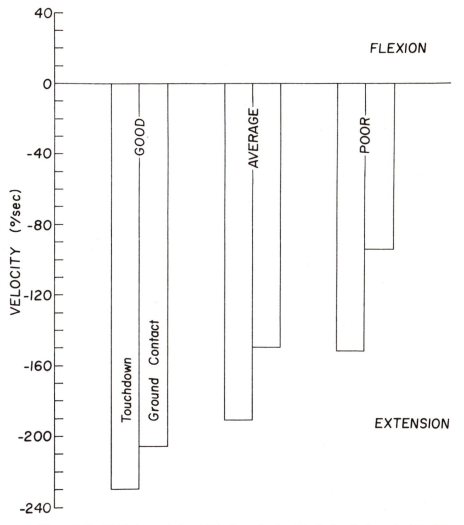

Figure 5.19. Thigh (upper leg) rotational speed going into the hurdle for male elite athlete 110-meter hurdlers.

at touchdown, the foot velocity is reduced, which further decreases the forward braking going into the hurdle. In addition, this action ensures that the lower leg is already moving toward the flexed position needed to begin the rapid extension required to drive

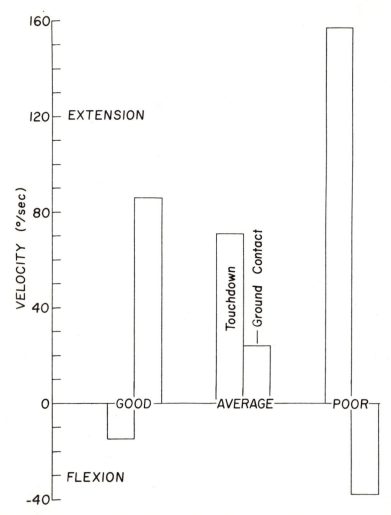

Figure 5.20. Leg (lower leg) rotational speed going into the hurdle for male elite athlete
110-meter hurdlers.

the body into the hurdle. Thus, during the final portion of the
ground phase, the lower leg should maximize extension speed.

Figures 5.19 and 5.20 indicate the upper- and lower-leg speed
going into the barrier for all elite athlete 110 hurdlers analyzed to
date. For comparison purposes, good, average, and poor values are
shown.

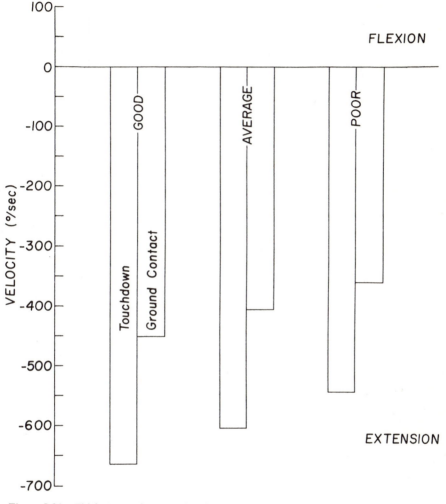

Figure 5.21. Thigh (upper leg) rotational speed coming off of the hurdle for male elite athlete 110-meter hurdlers.

Upper- and Lower-Leg Rotational Speed Coming off of the Hurdle (Individual Segment Result)

As in the stride going into the hurdle, the upper- and lower-leg speed coming off of the hurdle is of critical importance. Since this stride should be directed forward (not upward), there is no need to

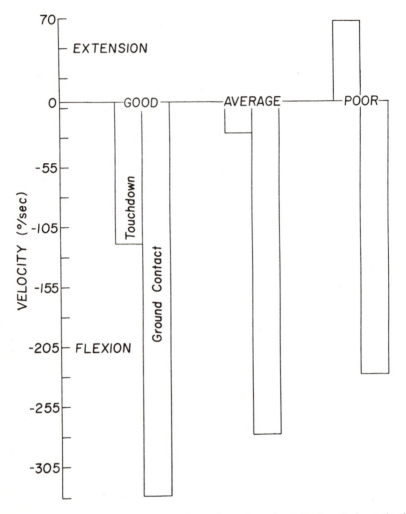

Figure 5.22. Leg (lower leg) rotational speed coming off of the hurdle for male elite athlete 110-meter hurdlers.

slow the body down. Thus the upper leg should land with high extension speed and should try to maintain the speed during ground contact. Since the upper leg is naturally extending at a high rate coming off of the hurdle, the speed cannot be totally maintained; however, the speed loss should be kept at a minimum.

The lower leg produces a very unusual motion during the ground phase coming off of the hurdle. At touchdown, as expected, the lower leg should be flexing to avoid horizontal braking. During ground contact, however, the lower leg should continue to flex. Since the body is coming down, off of the hurdle, the lower leg is attempting to pull the body toward the next stride. Since vertical speed is not needed during this stride, lower-leg extension is neither needed nor wanted. In the long hurdles, the need to produce a long stride after the hurdle may dictate modifying this action; however, lower leg extension should be initiated only after the body is well in front of the touchdown point.

Figures 5.21 and 5.22 present the upper- and lower-leg speeds coming off of the hurdle for male 110-meter hurdlers. For comparison, good, average, and poor values for each result, for all such performers investigated to date, are shown.

THE HURDLES: KINETIC RESULTS

As in sprinting, to actually measure the quality of the hurdling performance, the ground forces must be quantified. As the kinematic results point out, the critical movements are produced by the legs as they prepare for, or are actually involved in, ground contact both before and after the hurdle clearance. The following examples are for elite athlete female 100-meter hurdlers examined to date; except where noted, however, the trends can be expanded to apply to all hurdlers.

Vertical Force

Although hurdling appears to be a horizontal (forward) movement, the majority of the effort expended to negotiate the barrier is directed vertically (upward). Although vertical effort is critical in sprinting, since clearing the hurdle involves an exaggerated sprint stride with additional vertical emphasis, vertical effort appears to be even more critical in hurdling. Thus, a large vertical force is expected during ground contact going into the hurdler barrier. In addition, another large vertical force is needed to stop the performer's fall as touchdown occurs after the hurdle. Figure 5.23 shows the vertical ground forces produced by the elite athlete women short hurdle group before and after the hurdle. For comparison, values for good, average, and poor performance are indicated.

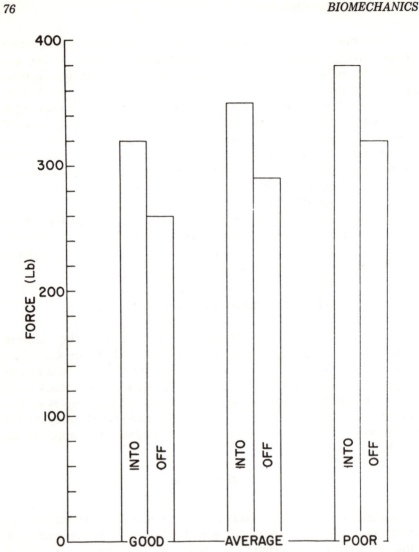

Figure 5.23. Vertical ground force going into and coming off of the hurdle for female elite athlete 100-meter hurdlers.

As indicated by Figure 5.23, the average vertical ground force is around 300 pounds. This is interesting since the average vertical force in sprinting is also around 300 pounds, and greater vertical effort is expected from the hurdlers. Thus, the questions become how the hurdlers get the additional vertical movement needed to clear the hurdle and how they minimize the force after the barrier. Both answers are related to how the performers alter the normal sprint stride to economize the amount of effort expended. Before the hurdle, the stride prior to hurdle clearance is shortened so that the body is not allowed to begin falling prior to ground contact. Thus, little or no vertical effort is needed to stop the downward fall of the hurdler, and it can all be used to project the body upward. In addition, going into the hurdle, the performer slightly extends the time on the ground, allowing a longer time for force production. After the hurdle, although the downward speed of the hurdler is large at impact, since the performer does not try to make the next stride long, a large vertical force is not needed to halt the fall and produce upward motion. Instead, the fall is halted, and only a small upward motion is produced as the stride off the hurdle is directed forward.

There are three additional productive ways to minimize the effects of the vertical force effort over the hurdle. The first is to minimize the weight of the performer by limiting the useless body fat and bulk a hurdler must carry. The second is to develop great leg strength in the performer so that the demands of the force are less fatiguing. Finally, proper body movements into, over, and after the hurdle can minimize the needed force, as well as modify any inefficient vertical force production generated during the movement.

Horizontal Force

Since a hurdler only wants to maintain maximum velocity, there is no need to produce any horizontal (forward and backward) force while on the ground. Unfortunately, to place the legs in a position to produce the necessary vertical force (Figure 5.23), unwanted horizontal force is produced which slows the body down during the first part of the ground phase. To maintain maximum horizontal velocity, therefore, the hurdler must produce a horizontal force in the opposite direction to speed up during the last portion of the ground phase. Figure 5.24 shows this pattern of negative (unwanted) force followed by positive (needed) force for all of the female elite athlete short hurdlers, both before and after the hurdle. For comparison, good, average, and poor results are indicated.

As Figure 5.24 indicates, the average horizontal forces in both directions are small compared to the vertical ground force (Figure 5.23). Since the negative horizontal force is unwanted and produced only because vertical force is needed, this force should be minimized. This can be done, without sacrificing the production of the needed

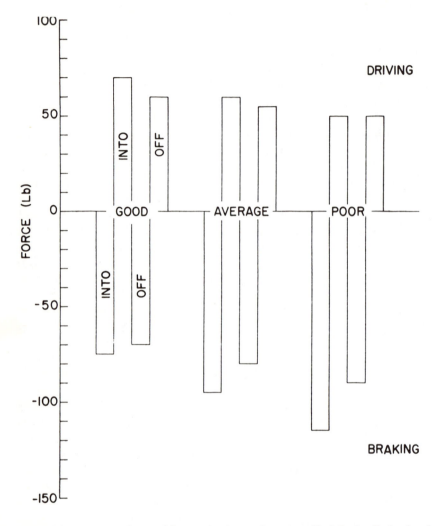

Figure 5.24. Horizontal ground force going into and coming off of the hurdle for female elite athlete 100-meter hurdlers.

vertical force, by using the hamstring and gluteal groups to pull the body over the touchdown leg during the first 20 to 30 percent of ground contact. This action demands great strength from a hurdler and is the cause of the majority of injuries sustained in hurdling. It is, however, the only way to economically produce the needed vertical force. Additionally, since an equal positive horizontal force is needed to offset the negative force, if the negative force is minimized, the amount of positive force needed to balance the negative force can be smaller. Figure 5.24 demonstrates both of these principles since the better performers produce less braking force and thus need less driving force to recover the lost speed. The results of Figure 5.24 also demonstrate that, during the ground phase before the hurdle, a large negative (unwanted) force is produced, which is not fully balanced by the positive (needed) force. Thus, hurdlers lose velocity going into the hurdle. After the hurdle, most of this lost speed is regained as the percentage of time that the positive force is being produced is much larger than the negative. The larger size of the negative force offsets some of the gain; however, the total effect of the ground phase after the hurdle is a net gain in horizontal velocity. Overall, a hurdler will lose speed while negotiating the barrier, although the better performers will minimize this loss.

If the hurdler does not possess sufficient leg strength, there is another way a hurdler can produce the necessary vertical force to negotiate the barrier. Vertical force can be easily produced by jamming the leg into the ground at touchdown, having the leg act as a pole vault pole, and vault the performer into the air. Unfortunately, this produces very high braking forces, which must be countered by very large positive forces during the second half of ground contact. This is, obviously, very energy wasteful and would severely reduce the endurance of the performance.

The horizontal force can be decreased by simply eliminating the potential to use the leg as a vaulting pole. By placing the leg under (instead of in front of) the body at touchdown, the leg cannot be used to produce the unwanted braking force. As mentioned previously, this is exactly the trend the better hurdlers are producing. Since this trend also decreases the vertical force production, the need for leg strength and precise technique is critical.

It is evident that the only direct way to effectively maximize the needed vertical force while minimizing the unwanted braking force is to produce the proper leg movement and develop and use large muscle forces in the legs. As in the vertical direction, horizontal force can be indirectly minimized, by reducing the weight (body fat and other unnecessary bulk) of the performer.

REFERENCES

1. Mann, R. V. *A comprehensive computer technique to process human motion data: Application to the flip long jump*. Microform Publications, College of Health, Physical Education and Recreation, University of Oregon, 1978.
2. Mann, R. V., and Sprague, P. A kinetic analysis of the ground leg in sprint running. *Research Quarterly for Exercise and Sport, 51*(2), May, 1980.
3. Mann, R. V. A kinetic analysis of sprinting. *Medicine and Science in Sports and Exercise, 13*(5), 1981.
4. Mann, R. V., and Sprague, P. The biomechanics of sprinting. *Biomechanics in Sports*, Academic Publishers, Del Mar, California, 1982.
5. Mann, R. V., and Sprague, P. The effects of muscular fatigue on the kinetics of sprint running. *Research Quarterly for Exercise and Sport, 54*(1), March, 1983.
6. Mann, R. V., Herman, J., Schultz, C., and Kotmel, J. A biomechanical analysis of elite sprint and hurdle athletes (Technical Reports 1-11). Colorado Springs, CO: Biomechanics Laboratory United States Olympic Training Center, 1982-1983.

CHAPTER **6**

Application of Biomechanical Principles: Optimization of Sport Technique

William Nelson

The application of biomechanical principles can be discussed in generalities or specifics. There has been much discussion over the years of how to optimize an athlete's technique. A general application of biomechanical principles concerns the various methods to optimize an athlete's technique. There are three main methods that are used by those involved with optimizing an athlete's technique.

A common method has been to follow a sequence of steps that lead to an optimization loop [1]. A typical qualitative loop used by most coaches consists of five steps:

1. Observe the performance.
2. Identify the technical factor that appears to limit the athlete's performance.
3. Interpret the meaning and significance of the identified limiting factor.
4. Establish an order of priority among the limiting factors.
5. Alter the athlete's technique based on the conclusion drawn from the analysis.

Figure 6.1 indicates the sequence of this loop arrangement.

The Elite Athlete, edited by N. K. Butts, T. T. Gushiken, and B. Zarins. Copyright © 1985 by Spectrum Publications, Inc.

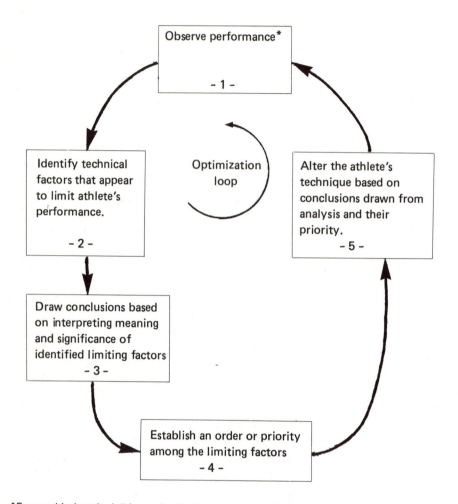

*For empirical method, "data collection" is used in lieu of "observe performance."

Figure 6.1. Optimization loop for sport technique.

The subjective nature of this method is a disadvantage; however, since it is probable that observation alone will not lead to identifying the limiting factors and could therefore lead to improper interpretation of the information.

Another method, commonly used by biomechanists, is an empirical method using sophisticated electronic equipment such as high speed cameras, digitizers, force platforms, and computers and applying digital filtering and statistical techniques to analyze the data and draw conclusions. The optimization loop for this method is similar to the first method except that data collection is used in lieu of observing performance. The empirical method used to analyze technique and performance could be used on a single group of subjects (correlation method) or on multiple groups (contrast method) of differing performance levels. Although the empirical method has significantly contributed to the wealth of information on technique and performance, it too has its limitations and disadvantages which include (1) the arbitrary manner in which the characteristics of the technique are selected to be analyzed often leads to important variables being omitted and/or irrelevant variables being included in the analysis, and (2) the sport technique used by the elite athlete may not be the best technique to use. This may lead to optimization of an inferior technique by concentrating on evolution of an old technique in lieu of innovation of a new technique.

A third method for identifying limiting factors of performance is the theoretical model method involving three basic steps [2]. They consist of:

1. The development of a theoretical model that relates the performance and the factors which produced that performance.
2. The collection and reduction of data on the performances of a large number of subjects whose ability extends over a wide range.
3. The evaluation of the data obtained in terms of the theoretical model.

The model is designed to provide a systematic basis for determining which biomechanical parameters to measure. A properly designed general model would include sufficient variables to identify the position and motion of the athlete from the moment the analysis begins. One major limitation of this method is the problem of multi-collinearity; however, several procedures exist that can be used to minimize its detrimental effects. Another problem of this method is the difficulty of explaining the results in terminology that is applicable to coaches and athletes.

PURPOSE

The analysis of most sports does not lend itself to convenient methods of collecting data. This poses an additional burden on the investigator. An investigator may have to forego the luxury of a laboratory setting in order to collect data under actual conditions during an athletic contest. The lack of accuracy of the environment that the investigator must use in an actual setting must be weighed against the lack of similarity in technique and level of performance an athlete might achieve in a laboratory simulation. Furthermore, the investigator must deal with providing coaches and athletes with the results of the analysis in a timely and effective manner using terminology that the coaches and athletes can understand and apply.

The purpose of this chapter is to describe how a multifaceted approach to utilizing the three methods of optimizing an athlete's technique can alleviate or minimize the disadvantage and short-comings of each method. In addition this chapter briefly addresses the problems the investigator faces in collecting and presenting data to the coaches and athletes in a timely and effective manner. To do this, the sport of rowing will be used as a specific example in the application of these methods of optimization.

ANALYSIS OF ROWING

In order to analyze properly a sport, a systematic approach must be developed that achieves the sport's overall biomechanical objectives. For rowing, as is usually the case, the overall objective is to provide the coach an additional tool to analyze individual athlete's technique and aid in development of the optimal technique for the athlete. Figure 6.2 depicts a flow chart that systematically indicates the steps required to achieve this objective. The flow chart can be broken up into two areas: (1) diagnostic and (2) prognostic [3]. The diagnostic section includes four main areas:

1. Basic factors of rowing.
2. Contrast actual rowing with rowing simulation.
3. Analysis of elite level athletes as a group.
4. Analysis of individual athletes.

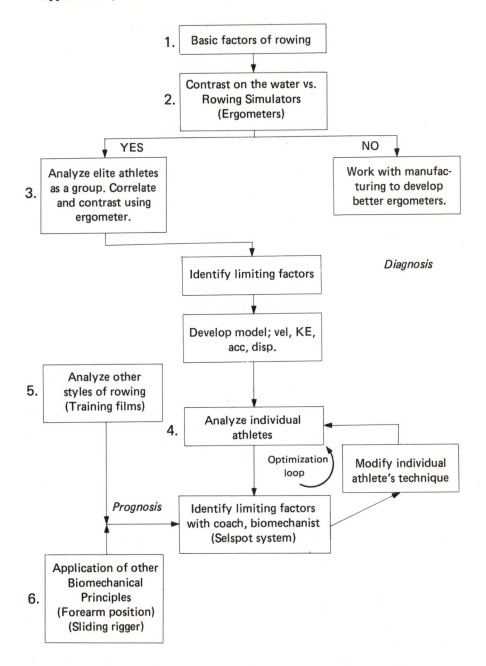

Figure 6.2. Flow chart for biomechanical analysis of rowing.

The prognostic section includes two other main areas:

5. Analysis of alternative styles of rowing.
6. Application of other biomechanical principles.

A more detailed explanation of each of these items will follow.

Basic Factors of Rowing

The basic factors of rowing can be broken down into many components (Figure 6.3) [4]. From this list, only those that directly relate to the biomechanics of the rower will be considered. From Figure 6.3, it can be seen that the force of the blade, angle of the oar, and time of pull are the only items related to the biomechanics of the rower. It is obvious that the analysis of the basic factors in rowing is based on the theoretical model method.

Contrast Actual Rowing with Rowing Simulation

Due to the difficulty and complexity of filming actual rowing regattas, the use of rowing ergometers is the obvious alternative. Also since physiological and pre-national team selection testing is commonly done on a rowing ergometer, it is important to know whether the various brands of rowing ergometers simulate actual rowing. This can easily be done by empirically contrasting actual rowing with ergometer rowing and determining if the athlete's body segments follow the same motion in each case.

Analysis of Elite-Level Athletes as a Group

Several different studies come under this general heading [5]. At the present time, they include: (a) National team members versus nonmembers, (b) male versus female, (c) effects of physiological fatigue on biomechanical factors, and (d) scullers versus sweep rowers. Each of these studies is directed at a specific situation that needs to be addressed before the limiting factors of the sport technique can be fully identified and understood.

A stick figure schematic is presented in Figure 6.4. Shown on the schematic are the basic biomechanical parameters that are used in the analysis. A summary of the various derived biomechanical parameters and their significance is presented in Table 6.1. The empirical method is used in this phase of the flow chart. Both the

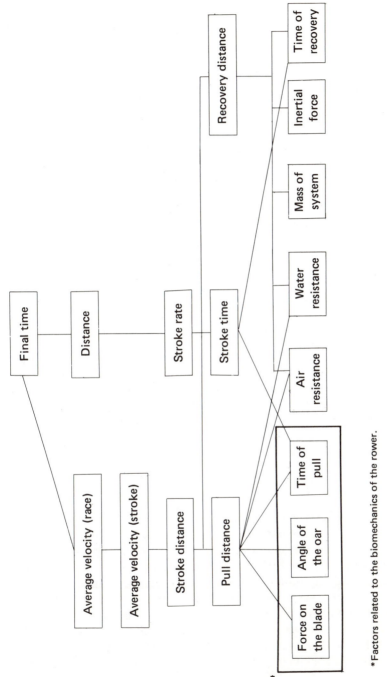

*Factors related to the biomechanics of the rower.

Figure 6.3. Basic factors in rowing [4].

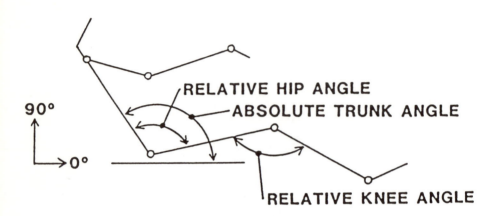

Figure 6.4. Stick figure schematic of rowing.

correlation and contrast is used depending on which specific study is referenced. It can be easily understood how the limitation expressed earlier with the empirical method apply in this situation. Even though thirteen separate characteristics were analyzed, it would be presumptuous to suggest that all of the significant biomechanical parameters are included. A review of Table 6.1 quickly suggests that there are several irrelevant parameters included.

Analysis of Individual Athletes

Once the analysis of elite level athletes as a group is complete, and the limiting factors have been identified, these factors, combined with prognostic biomechanical information, can then by applied to the individual athlete to determine his/her limiting factors. This is the beginning of the individual's optimization loop which involves input from many sources, especially the athlete's coach. It is at this point that the biomechanist must work closely with the coach, who may have determined from experience what he/she considers is the "best" rowing style. In this situation, the biomechanist may find himself/herself in an advisory position to help the coach quantify in lieu of

Table 6.1. ANOVA Results

	$\overline{X}$	±SD	$\overline{X}$	±SD	F Ratio	P<
1-min ergometer score (rpm)	431	21.0	521	37.2	37.0	0.01
Height (m)	1.70	0.04	1.75	0.04	5.53	0.05
Weight (kg)	68.45	9.04	70.37	6.10	0.29	N.S.
Oar velocity when perp. to shell (m·s^{-1})	2.17	0.19	2.58	0.21	18.77	0.01
Maximum angular kinetic energy of legs and trunk (J)	11.43	2.44	14.88	4.85	3.35	N.S.
Angular kinetic energy of legs and trunk when perp. to shell (J)	9.00	3.20	12.14	4.14	3.12	N.S.
Time between oar perp. and maximum angular kinetic energy (s)	0.175	0.089	0.136	0.045	1.48	N.S.
Angular velocity of trunk when oar perp. to shell (rad·s^{-1})	2.85	0.68	3.13	0.46	1.07	N.S.
Angular velocity of knee when oar perp. to shell (rad·s^{-1})	3.01	0.96	4.18	0.48	11.51	0.01
Time between oar perp. and maximum angular velocity of trunk (s)	0.083	0.039	0.060	0.021	2.44	N.S.
Sum of knee and trunk angular velocity when oar perp. (rad·s^{-1})	5.86	0.61	7.31	0.76	19.37	0.01
Time between maximum angular velocity of knee and trunk (s)	0.235	0.049	0.150	0.061	10.36	0.01
Efficiency (%)	75.8	10.10	87.2	6.88	8.18	0.05

Nonselected (N=8), Selected (N=10)

modifying the coach's particular style of rowing. One of the coach's and athlete's main concern at this stage is to obtain the results of the analysis as soon as possible. In response to this concern, a rapid portable data analysis system is being developed using a personal computer and SelCom sensing camera that allows almost instantaneous turnaround. This permits the coach to monitor changes in the

Table 6.2. Summary of Flow Chart Items and Applicable Analysis Method

Flow Chart Item	Analysis Method		
	Observation	Empirical Correlation/Contrast	Theoretical Model
1. Basic factors of rowing			*
2. Actual versus ergometer rowing		*	
3. Analyze elite athletes as a group			
(a) National team members versus nonmembers		*	
(b) Male versus female		*	
(c) Effects of physiological fatigue		*	
(d) Scullers versus sweep rowers		*	
4. Analyze individual athletes			
(a) Selspot system	*	*	
5. Analyze other style of rowing			
(a) Training films	*		
6. Other biomechanical principles			
(a) Forearm position on oar		*	
(b) Sliding rigger	*	*	*

athlete's rowing style quantitatively as well as by observation. Any number of parameters may be programmed into the computer that the coach, biomechanist, and/or athlete would like to see.

Analysis of Alternative Styles of Rowing

In most cases, this is done qualitatively by observing films taken of crews during racing situations. The crews are filmed at high speed which allow for a more thorough subjective analysis.

Application of Other Biomechanical Principles

This category pertains to innovative ideas which are developed using general biomechanical principles and applying them to a specific sport. Two items within this category include (1) the forearm position relative to the oar handle [6] and (2) the sliding rigger in lieu of the sliding seat. Again, the development of ideas in this category requires cooperation between biomechanists, coaches and, possibly equipment manufacturers. Depending on the particular item, any one or combination of the three methods of analysis could be used.

SUMMARY

A summary of the major components of the flow chart and the corresponding method(s) of analysis is listed in Table 6.2. The analysis of sport technique is complex and requires innovative ideas, methods, and compromises if the investigator is to be successful and make a contribution to the understanding and development of an efficient sport technique. As can be seen from the example of rowing, each situation requires considerable thought and discussion as to what will be sacrificed and/or gained if a particular method of analysis is chosen. It is hoped that new methods of analysis will be developed and a better application of the limitations and uses of existing methods will permit more accurate and applicable biomechanic research in the future.

REFERENCES

1. Borysiewicz, M., Bucks, J., and Komor, A. Optimization of sport techniques using the example of weight lifting. In *Biomechanics VII B* (pp. 305-312). Baltimore, MD: University Park Press, 1981.

2. Hay, J. G., Vaughan, C. L., and Woodworth, G. G. Techniques and performance: Identifying the limiting factors. In *Biomechanics VII B* (pp. 511-520). Baltimore, MD: University Park Press, 1981.

3. Bober, T. Biomechanical aspects of sports techniques. In *Biomechanics VII B* (pp. 501-510). Baltimore, MD: University Park Press, 1981.

4. Schneider, E., and Hauser, M. Biomechanical analysis of performances in rowing. In *Biomechanics VII B* (pp. 431-435). Baltimore, MD: University Park Press, 1981.

5. Nelson, W., and Widule, C. Biomechanics: New frontiers of rowing. *Rowing U.S.A.*, *15*(2), 23-27, 1983.

6. Bompa, T. O. Elbow flexor muscles effectiveness in sagittal plane, employing different forearm positions. In A. Ayalon (Ed.), *Biomechanics of sport games and sport activities* (pp. 66-71). Israel: Wingate Institute, 1979.

CHAPTER 7

The Teaching of Biomechanics: How to Educate Coaches

Keith French

Sports participation is recognized by many as a meaningful activity. If this assumption is valid, then, according to Nelson, scientific efforts designed for the improvement of sports performance are equally worthwhile. Of the many subdisciplines of what has come collectively to be called sports science—biomechanics, exercise science, sport psychology, and sport sociology—which are directed specifically toward the improvement of human performance, perhaps none has greater potential than biomechanics [1].

Biomechanics is defined by Cooper as, " . . . the study of the mechanics of living organisms (man) especially under conditions of sudden, violent or prolonged strain such as experienced in sports" [2]. Nelson favors a definition of sport biomechanics to emphasize the specific application to sport skills that is recognized worldwide [3]. Regardless of the definition, the biomechanical study of human motion is accomplished only through the application of mechanical principles in combination with a knowledge of the anatomical and physiological characteristics of the performer.

Biomechanics has grown rapidly as a mode of scientific inquiry. Common applications for biomechanical principles and concepts include space science, automobile safety, orthopedic surgery,

The Elite Athlete, edited by N. K. Butts, T. T. Gushiken, and B. Zarins. Copyright © 1985 by Spectrum Publications, Inc.

biomedical engineering, physical rehabilitation, and more recently sports performance [4]. Several significant biomechanical contributions have been made to sports performance: the quantification of a variety of sport skills, the description of skill execution techniques, the identification of fundamental principles, the clarification of controversies in the subjective analysis of sport skills, and the influence on the design and construction of sports equipment [1].

Physical educators have long assumed that an awareness of the mechanisms of movement will better equip and prepare learners to learn, teachers to teach, and coaches to detect and correct errors in sports performance [5]. Unfortunately, there is little evidence to support the contention that a knowledge of biomechanics is essential for the performer. Many world-class athletes know very little about biomechanics. The teacher/coach, on the other hand, requires a thorough knowledge of biomechanics that is derived from other than personal performance experiences [6]. It can safely be assumed that teachers and coaches need to be well informed about biomechanical principles to effectively present correct skill techniques and to be able to identify incorrect movement fundamentals. No longer is it sufficient for them to simply describe a sport skill in terms of how it felt to them when they performed the movement [1].

With a recognized need established for the education of coaches in biomechanics, attention will now be focused on how the educational process might be accomplished. Both formal and informal processes will be presented.

HOW TO EDUCATE COACHES IN BIOMECHANICS

The goal of education in biomechanics, as identified by Lissner, is to provide basic information that will enhance communication between individuals from different disciplines, enabling them to maximize their specific contribution to a combined effort [7]. In the education of coaches, this goal establishes the need to develop a fundamental knowledge of biomechanical principles which will permit communication between coaches and scientists so that relevant performance information may be applied at the practical level.

Until fairly recently, the efforts to scientifically educate coaches have been limited mainly to undergraduate programs in physical education, with little evidence that these programs have been very successful in promoting relevance to teaching or coaching.

One of the major problems in teaching biomechanics is to educate the teachers in the professional preparation programs so that they will teach meaningfully. It has become increasingly apparent that the primary interpretation role between the researcher and the practitioner must be filled by those who teach in the coaching preparation programs. They must condense and simplify biomechanical information so that future coaches will become accustomed to the practical application of such information.

Several levels of coaching may be recognized, each presenting a unique challenge to the educational effort:

1. Youth sport or volunteer coaches
2. Middle and secondary school coaches
3. College and university coaches
4. Professional coaches
5. National amateur sport coaches

In addition, consideration should be given to whether the coach is involved with individual or team sports. Individual sport coaches are inclined to be more receptive to education and research. Perhaps it is the preoccupation with strategy that causes team sport coaches to be more resistant to scientific information.

Being practically oriented, coaches are not always as intellectually curious about why or how something works as the scientist may be. Often they simply are satisfied with knowing something will work. Not infrequently this may lead to the misapplication of mechanical principles, e.g., the concept of power as traditionally applied in weight training ignores the rate of force application that is required in the mechanical definition.

Regardless of their level of coaching or personal philosophy, it is evident that coaches need to receive better education to enable them to make greater and more practical use of biomechanical information. Time is the major limitation for coaches. If they lack a sound initial background, there is unlikely to be sufficient time to adequately correct the problem once they begin coaching.

Nelson indicated two primary ways for teachers and coaches to overcome deficiencies in biomechanical knowledge: (1) in-service or continuing education, such as clinics and workshops, for those already in the professional field; and (2) upgrading of both undergraduate and graduate curricular offerings [1]. Thus, education in biomechanics can be accomplished formally or informally through pre-service or in-service programs, with the former being the preferred method.

Formal Preparation

Formal preparation includes any organized training that a coach receives, either prior to beginning an active coaching role or as a supplement to it. Normally such training is intended to meet minimum standards of expertise, occurs in a customary educational setting, and earns credit toward a degree. Typical examples are coaching concentration and/or certification programs which are designed to satisfy entrance level requirements only.

Originally, formal training was offered at the undergraduate level and was most often limited to physical education majors. Today, most undergraduate physical education programs offer coaching concentrations, perhaps with certification, to nonmajors as well. Graduate-level programs and programs for the preparation of volunteer coaches are becoming more common too.

The initial obstacle encountered at the undergraduate level is the lack of a common curriculum [8]. Biomechanists have failed to reach agreement as to which courses to include, in addition to biomechanics or traditional kinesiology. Cooper suggested that minimal preparation must include some knowledge of anatomy, mathematics, and physics along with detailed understanding of at least one sport. Adrian favored a more holistic approach, giving equal time to physics and biology. Other courses that might be included are computer science, motor learning, and physiology [9].

Since the majority of coaches still receive their formal training in schools of physical education, it seems logical to examine those curricula in more detail. A national survey of existing kinesiology programs, for the National Conference on the Undergraduate Teaching of Kinesiology held at the University of Illinois in June 1977, found that both anatomical and mechanical considerations were emphasized along with an application to movement analysis [10].

The Guidelines and Standards for Undergraduate Kinesiology, developed in 1980 by the Kinesiology Academy of the National Association for Sport and Physical Education, identified the purpose for studying undergraduate kinesiology as being twofold: (1) to provide students with the necessary knowledge to systematically analyze motor skills; and (2) to provide experience in the application of that knowledge to the execution and evaluation of both the performer and the performance. Prerequisites in anatomy and mathematics were emphasized as necessary for the development of adequate anatomical, mechanical and application competencies [11].

Another point of controversy concerns the methodology employed to teach the mechanics of human movement. Should a quantitative or qualitative emphasis be used? Again, biomechanicians are not in total agreement. Those who are more theoretically oriented may tend to favor a quantitative approach while those with a practical orientation will more likely be inclined toward a qualitative emphasis.

Norman makes a strong case for a qualitative approach. In his approach, a series of basic biomechanical principles are applied during the visual analysis of human movement. It is assumed that the violation of one or more of the following principles is the cause of errors in most performances [8].

1. Summation of joint torques
2. Continuity of joint torques
3. Impulse
4. Reaction
5. Equilibrium
6. Summation and continuity of body segment velocities
7. Generation of angular momentum
8. Conservation of momentum
9. Moment of inertia manipulation
10. Body segment angular momentum manipulation

The first step in Norman's approach is to identify the mechanical purpose or objective of the movement, as opposed to the performance purpose. The former is the cause of the movement while the latter is simply the desired outcome. The second step is to identify errors in the performance in relation to violations of the above biomechanical principles [8].

The major benefits derived from Norman's approach are (1) a minimum background is required in mechanics, lessening the need for a complicated terminology; (2) students may apply the biomechanical principles without extensive quantitative measurements or calculations; (3) the impossible task of memorization of "how-to-do-it" manuals is eliminated; and (4) students learn the practical application of biomechanics and not just about biomechanics [8].

Similar methods of qualitative analysis are advocated by Hay and Reid [12] and Kreigbaum and Barthels [13]. The Guidelines and Standards for Undergraduate Kinesiology also support the qualitative approach, recommending a minimum of quantitative methodology to develop an understanding of fundamental concepts, with the major emphasis on the practical application of qualitative knowledge to the evaluation of human movement [11].

It has been this author's experience that the typical undergraduate student lacks a sufficient background in mathematics and physics to handle a comprehensive quantitative analysis. Therefore, the qualitative method should be stressed at the undergraduate level with the techniques of analysis receiving considerable attention during the preparation of teachers or coaches.

Hoffman presented a three-level model for the training of teachers/coaches involving observation, evaluation, and diagnosis. Observation, the most frequently used coaching technique, is often the most poorly developed. Observational skill cannot simply be assumed; formal experience with observational techniques must be provided. The notion that performance skill facilitates observation lacks sufficient supporting evidence. Cognitive knowledge of the skill may be just as important [4].

Evaluation requires that judgments be made about the correctness of the performance, in terms of accuracy and specificity. A clear understanding of mechanical principles is necessary to appropriately evaluate a skill. This knowledge comes from both practical performance experiences and the cognitive application of mechanical principles. Hoffman pointed out that a major obstacle to the skill analysis training of teachers/coaches is the lack of a taxonomy of common sports performance [14].

Diagnosis is the most difficult proficiency to develop. Since the cause of the error is often far removed from the visible effect, an accurate interpretation can be made only through the application of biomechanical principles. Hoffman doubts if a generic facility for diagnosis can be developed. A stock supply of biomechanical principles is no assurance of a correct analysis; rather teachers/ coaches must be provided with learning experiences that will facilitate their diagnostic development [14].

There are relatively few graduate programs in biomechanics directed specifically toward the development of coaches. However, Kelly and Luttgens reported, from a collection of opinions about the standards and guidelines for gradurate programs in biomechanics, that coaching was an appropriate subspecialization or concentration at the master's level [15]. Cooper cited the master's degree program in the theory of coaching at Lakehead University as an innovative program designed to meet the particular needs of senior, national, and international coaches. The focus is on the three basic sciences of biomechanics, physiology, and psychology as they relate to the performance of elite athletes [16].

In summary, the writer believes that the formal education of coaches should parallel that of physical educators in terms of scientific background with the addition of coaching theory classes and a coaching practicum. Biomechanical principles and analysis techniques should be presented qualitatively. As Huelster pointed out, it is futile to expect teachers and coaches to memorize the skills of all of the sports to which they are going to be exposed [17].

Prospective coaches, like teachers, need to have extensive analysis experiences to learn to distinguish between the real errors of performance and the symptoms of errors. Nonspecific or pet error corrections should be discouraged.

The difference between a technique and style needs to be clarified. A technique is the application of a mechanical principle during the execution of a skill. Style is the nonessential or personal application of mechanical principles, e.g., the number of preliminary swings before driving a golf ball. A technique is not wrong unless it violates a mechanical principle.

Informal Preparation

Informal preparation includes those experiences that a coach has that are shorter term in nature, usually without educational credit, and often less well organized. Some of the experiences may occur prior to the beginning of active coaching, but most will occur afterward. Examples of informal preparation are preliminary playing experience; on-the-job training; attendance at clinics, symposia, or workshops; and the reading of performance-related publications.

Preliminary playing experience is the most basic preparation that a coach may have. While it is assumed to be essential by many coaches, it unfortunately does not guarantee success in coaching. There are perhaps as many successful coaches with limited playing experience as there are unsuccessful coaches with considerable experience. The major benefit to be derived from playing experience is a broader knowledge of the particular sport. Playing experience, coupled with on-the-job training is the most common background for coaches. Neither relates particularly well to biomechanics, however.

Clinics and symposia can become valuable sources of biomechanical information for coaches with some modification of the usual format. Traditionally, clinics have presented "how-to" material which translated into variations in technique rather than true biomechanical principles. Biomechanists have to be urged to present their papers and research findings, in a qualitative manner, directly to the coaches at their clinics. While this is happening more frequently now than in the past, further encouragement is still necessary. Coaches, on the other hand, ought to consider attending bio-mechanical symposia to at least become somewhat acquainted with the quantitative data that may be presented in their particular sport.

The programs designed to train youth sport and community coaches are good examples of informal workshop preparation. By definition, youth sport or community coaches are those volunteers who work at other occupations and coach in the evenings or on weekends. Traditionally, they lack formal education in coaching and come from varied backgrounds of sport experience. Most youth sport coaches have depended upon playing experience, on-the-job training, or attendance at an occasional clinic for their coaching knowledge. They rarely possess expertise in biomechanics.

Norman described the program used to educate community coaches in Canada, where more coaching is done by community coaches than by physical educators. With government support, scientific material has been added to traditional clinic presenta-tions. University faculty specialists, all with previous university coaching experience, serve as instructors in sport psychology, growth and development, sports medicine, biomechanics, motor learning, and work physiology. The biomechanics portion consists of three levels: (1) Level I—introduction to biomechanical princi-ples with an emphasis on error detection; (2) Level II—qualitative analysis techniques applied to the actual performance of peers; and (3) Level III—application of biomechanical principles to measurement methods [18].

The most ambitious and successful program for the education of youth sports personnel in the United States is provided by the Youth Sports Institute of Michigan State University, under the direction of Dr. Vern Seefeldt. Established by the state legislature, this program has a three-fold purpose: (1) to provide in-service education for nonschool youth sports coaches, (2) to produce educational materials suitable for the needs of volunteer coaches, and (3) to conduct research concerning the potential beneficial or detrimental effects of competitive athletics on children and youth. The educational offerings consist of introductory and leadership programs for coaches and a program for sports directors. Over 15,000 coaches, parents, and sports administrators have taken part in these workshops [19].

The success of the Canadian and Michigan State programs suggest that volunteer coaches can and do understand biomechanical principles and concepts when scientific jargon is minimized and complex principles are simplified and transformed into practical applications. It seems reasonable to expect that full-time coaches, with a more sound initial preparation, can profit equally well from such experiences. The key is to provide qualitative information in a terminology that coaches readily understand and will accept.

Apparently, there is a universal problem of inadequate communication between the researcher and the practitioner. Dillman said that the biomechanics researcher frequently lacks an understanding of sports and their execution; he has a good theory base but no practical base. Conversely, the coach does not readily understand the research process; he has a good practical base but a limited theory base [20].

Presenting coaches with research findings that may be applied at the practical level involves problems of both communication and interpretation. Nelson suggested that even though scientific knowledge is available, there is still a problem in delivering meaningful information to coaches and athletes. Athletes often become suspicious after they are used as subjects for research and then receive no feedback [3]. Mazur noted, following a series of interviews with coaches, trainers, and athletes, that the lag in the implementation of new methods is often due to the feeling that some scientists are more interested in publishing than in sincerely addressing performance problems [21].

Cooper emphasized that teachers and coaches must first become convinced of the practical value of research findings. Often they are turned off by theoretical emphases and research lingo. The researcher has the responsibility to interpret more carefully his results in the language of the coaches. By following the European lead, in which research is conducted after a need has been established in a specific area, the sincerity of the research effort may be more readily accepted [2].

Serial publications provide the best immediate source of biomechanical information for the coach. There is, however, a serious dichotomy in the available publications that must be recognized. Coaching literature is filled with biomechanical errors; biomechanical literature is not written with the real consumers (coaches and athletes) in mind. A substantial effort will be required to overcome these conflicting conditions. Biomechanists must be urged to publish their research findings in the non-technical journals that coaches routinely read, knowingly risking credit from their institutions for publishing in a nonrefereed publication. Coaches will need considerable encouragement before they can be expected to read regularly the more technical research publications.

The nontechnical, teacher/coach-oriented publications include:

> *Coaching: Women's Athletics*
> *International Gymnast*
> *Journal of Physical Education, Recreation and Dance*
> *Physician and Sports Medicine*
> *Runner's World*
> *Scholastic Coach*
> *Swimming Technique*
> *The Athletic Journal*
> *Track and Field Technique*
> *Women's Varsity Sports* [22]

Among the more technical, research-oriented journals are the following:

> *American Journal of Sports Medicine*
> *Canadian Journal of Applied Sport Sciences*
> *International Journal of Sports Medicine*
> *Journal of Biomechanics*
> *Journal of Human Movement Studies*
> *Journal of Sports Medicine and Physical Fitness*
> *Motor Skills: Theory Into Practice*
> *Medicine and Science in Sports and Exercise*
> *Research Quarterly for Exercise and Sport*
> *Scandinavian Journal of Sports Sciences* [22]

Each applied organization and federation is developing its own publication for specific interests. Following are some of the special publications and proceedings of conferences held by the professional associations:

> *American College of Sports Medicine Bulletin*
> *American Society of Biomechanics Newsletter*
> *Biomechanics I–VII: International Series on Sport Sciences*

> *Completed Research in Health, Physical Education and*
>   *Recreation*
> *Exercise and Sport Science Reviews*
> *International Society of Biomechanics Newsletter*
> *Kinesiology Academy Newsletter*
> *Swimming I, II, III: International Series on Sport Sciences*
> *What Research Tells the Coach: AAHPERD Series in Various*
>   *Sports* [22]

Nelson identified the need for a scientific publication that is exclusively devoted to sport biomechanics. The purpose of such a publication would be to collate research that is currently being published in a variety of other journals. Extensive communication benefits would result from this journal for all of those interested in sports performance [23].

The establishment of the Education Services Department for Sports Medicine by the United States Olympic Committee, which can provide library or information retrieval services, is a very important step in bridging the communication gap between biomechanists and coaches. Now coaches must be convinced and educated to use the service. Similar but smaller operations might be established at other sites. Abstract services, in the form of a newsletter, from these operations could be invaluable for keeping the busy coach up-to-date in his sport.

The informal methods of clinics, workshops, and publications offer numerous opportunities to update coaches with biomechanical information. No single method is superior; alert coaches will take advantage of all occasions to keep themselves informed of new developments in their sport. While it is the formal preparation in qualitative biomechanics that lays the groundwork, it is the informal methods that enable coaches to stay current. To be truly effective and well prepared, coaches must use both preparations.

Education in biomechanics has an exciting potential for growth. Coaches are becoming increasingly familiar with biomechanical evaluation techniques; their ability to analyze the mechanics of sports has grown dramatically in recent years. As a result, the gap between scientific needs and athletic habits has narrowed considerably [21]. With more scientific training methods, a true appreciation for the value of biomechanics will be developed.

REFERENCES

1. Nelson, R. C. Contributions of biomechanics to improved human performance. Paper presented at the American Academy of Physical Education, Milwaukee, WI, 1976.
2. Cooper, J. M. Reaction paper presented at the American Academy of Physical Education, Milwaukee WI, 1976.
3. Nelson, R. C. From kinesiology to sport biomechanics. Paper presented at AAHPERD Convention, Minneapolis MN, 1983.
4. Miller, D. I., and Nelson, R. C. *Biomechanics of Sport*, Philadelphia: Lea and Febiger, 1973.
5. Locke, L. F. Kinesiology and the profession, *JOHPER*, September 1965, 69-71.
6. Burke, R. K. Relationships in physical education: A viewpoint from biomechanics. Paper presented at the American Academy of Physical Education, Seattle, 1977.
7. Lissner, H. R. Biomechanics—What is it? Paper presented at the winter annual meeting of the American Society of Mechanical Engineers, New York, 1962.
8. Norman, R. W. An approach to teaching the mechanics of human motion at the undergraduate level. In C. J. Dillman and R. G. Sears (Eds.), *Proceedings Kinesiology: A National Conference on Teaching.* Urbana-Champaign, IL: University of Illinois, 1977.
9. Adrian, M. J. The true meaning of biomechanics. In J. M. Cooper and B. Haven (Eds.), *Biomechanics Symposium Proceedings.* Bloomington, IN: Indiana University, 1980.
10. Deutsch, H., et al. Present status of kinesiology: Results of a national survey. In C. J. Dillman and R. G. Sears (Eds.), *Proceedings Kinesiology: A National Conference on Teaching.* Urbana-Champaign, IL: University of Illinois, 1977.
11. Guidelines and standards for undergraduate kinesiology, *JOPER*, February 1980, 19-21.
12. Hay, J. G., and Reid, J. G. *The Anatomical and Mechanical Bases of Human Motion.* Englewood Cliffs, NJ: Printice-Hall, Inc., 1982.
13. Kreighbaum, E., and Barthels, K. M. *Biomechanics: A Qualitative Approach for Studying Human Movement.* Minneapolis, MN: Burgess Publishing Co., 1981.
14. Hoffman, S. J. Toward taking the fun out of skill analysis. *JOHPER*, November-December, 1974, 74-76.
15. Kelley, D. L., and Luttgens, K. Investigating guidelines and standards for graduate programs in biomechanics. In J. M. Cooper and B. Haven (Eds.), *Biomechanics Symposium Proceedings*, Bloomington, IL: Indiana University, 1980.
16. Cooper, J. M. Biomechanics. In M. L. Krotee (Ed.), Cross-cultural dimensions of scientific inquiry, *JOPER*, November/December, 1980, 43-44.
17. Huelster, L. J. Learning to analyze performance. *JOHPER*, 1939, 10, 84, 120-121.

18. Norman, R. W. Biomechanics for the community coach. *JOPER*, March 1975, 46, 3, 49-52.
19. Youth Sports Institute. Educational programs for coaches and sports managers. East Lansing, MI: Michigan State University, 1981.
20. Dillman, C. J. Personal communication, September 29, 1983.
21. Mazur, S. Winners. *Omni*, July 1980, 2, 45-46.
22. Kreighbaum, E., and Barthels, K. M. *Instructor's Supplement to Biomechanics: A Qualitative Approach for Studying Human Movement*, Minneapolis, MN: Burgess Publishing Co., 1981.
23. Nelson, R. C. Biomechanics: Past and present. In J. M. Cooper and B. Haven (Eds.), *Biomechanics Symposium Proceedings*, Bloomington, IL: Indiana University, 1980.

CHAPTER 8

The Need for Interdisciplinary Research in Sports Science

Charles J. Dillman

During the last several years, we have witnessed a phenomenal growth within the total field of sports science. Based upon some excellent and creative research conducted within the areas of sports medicine, physiology, biomechanics, and psychology, we have gained an understanding of the many unique phenomena that occur when individuals participate in sports activities. For example, researchers in biomechanics have finally moved away from worrying about how they could quantify motion to the nearest micrometer to actually solving problems and making recommendations for the improvement of performance. Recent technical developments now enable biomechanists to provide athletes with immediate results whereas several years ago it took at least six months for a project to be completed.

While this progress is the result of many dedicated scientists, I would like to suggest that all is not well within the field of sports science. It is my opinion that there is a major weakness in sports science, and this deficiency stems from the lack of integration of ideas and problem solving both within various disciplines and among areas. Thus, I believe that until a concerted effort is made to form interdisciplinary teams, the field of sports science will stagnate and not produce effective solutions for many problems.

To illustrate the need for integration of knowledge and ideas, I have selected several examples from the area of biomechanics. The initial case will indicate a successful solution to a problem due to the work of an interdisciplinary team while the other examples will delineate the necessity for interdisciplinary research.

OPTIMIZATION OF PERFORMANCE

One of the major objectives of sports biomechanics is to optimize the performance of a given athlete. Theoretically, with respect to the physical morphology and capabilities of each individual, there exists an optimum manner in which to perform a skill. Finding this ideal or optimal performance for individual athletes is still a very difficult problem. At the present time, for most sports skills, there are no theoretical solutions available which can provide a true optimal analysis of an individual performance.

Present biomechanical evaluations are generally conducted by comparing an athlete's style to the best in the world. The assumption of these comparative analyses is that elite athletes through years and years of practice have optimized their performance and that their techniques can serve as criteria in the evaluation of skill. In addition, some theoretical interpretation and justification of results are made by applying the laws of mechanics to explain why a certain maneuver is better than others.

An example of this type of evaluation is illustrated by a recent project conducted by our research group on the influence of biomechanical factors upon the speed of ice-hockey players. A review of literature revealed that a multiple regression model had already been developed [1] that related selected biomechanical factors to acceleration capacity of ice-hockey players. Utilizing and validating this model in the evaluation of amateur hockey players led us to the conclusion that speed could be improved if the leg extension phase were performed from a more flexed position. This group of high-level hockey players seemed to accelerate from a very upright position. A more technical interpretation of these results indicated that if these hockey players exerted more of the available force in the desired direction of motion, this ability to accelerate would improve.

While this type of analysis and resultant findings are useful to skating coaches in trying to improve technique, they are not truly optimal solutions for individual athletes. Fortunately, however, as the field of sports biomechanics has progressed, there has been an increased interest in finding solutions to optimizing human performance. One of the leaders in this area is Dr. Herbert Hatze from the University of Vienna in Austria. Over a period of ten years, Dr. Hatze and his strong interdisciplinary research team have worked in developing a total system for the optimization of human movement using optimal control theory.

In a recent article, Dr. Hatze [2] relates the successful optimization of the long-jump event. Prior to the optimization, an athlete had an average performance of 6.58 meters with his longest jump ever of 6.96 meters. Via computer simulation and optimization techniques, Hatze was able to determine the ideal performance pattern for this athlete. Graphical techniques were employed to compare the optimized jump with normal performance to facilitate the identification of errors. The main discrepancy in performance was an insufficient and delayed extension of the hip joint at takeoff. After three weeks of correcting this and other errors, the athlete's *average* performance increased to 7.12 meters (an improvement of 46 centimeters!).

The point of this example is that a major contribution to the field of biomechanics is being made as a result of teamwork by experts from various areas. These optimization problems are so complex that it takes an effort by a group consisting of system engineers, researchers, numerical mathematicians, computer programmers, and optimal control specialists to solve the problem. Hatze explains that work along these lines is continuing and he feels (perhaps over-optimistically) that within a few years computerized optimization of sports motions will be performed quite frequently. It seems to follow that if the biomechanics area can benefit from this type of integration surely all other subdisciplines within sports science such as physiology, psychology, and motor integration could accelerate their advancement by encouraging more interdisciplinary work within their respective areas.

With the progress attained over the last few years plus advancements toward optimizing performance, the area of biomechanics is now providing specific guidelines for the improvement of technique. However, the remaining problem is, How do we get this information into practice? In a number of cases, effective implementation depends upon utilizing the resources and expertise of other disciplines. Figure 8.1 illustrates how biomechanics might relate to four other broad areas within sports science. The following problems and examples describe how biomechanics would benefit from interaction with these separate areas to facilitate the implementation of information and improvement of performance.

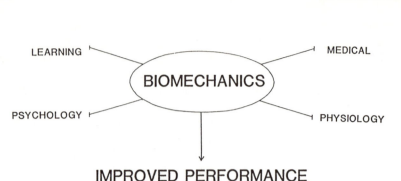

Figure 8.1. Relationship of biomechanics to other areas of sports science.

Race Walking

At the Olympic Training Center we have been conducting ground reaction force studies with resident race walkers. During one of these force platform investigations, it was observed that an athlete had some asymmetry between left and right legs. This difference was particularly apparent upon reviewing the front-to-back force patterns. Figure 8.2 illustrates these differences between right and left feet. Note that with the right foot there is a brief decelerating force (negative values in Figure 8.2) followed by an accelerating force (positive values are directed forward). On the left foot, the duration of the decelerating force (acting backward with respect to body) is significantly longer, and the accelerating force (acting in the direction of motion) is much lower and acts over a shorter period than observed with the right foot. This athlete seems to be moving over the ground by propulsive forces exerted by the right foot. This asymmetry between right and left legs was also very noticeable on the high-speed films synchronized with the force platform record-ings. The obvious question is, How does the athlete correct this problem?

After having tried several corrections such as "don't lock the knee before contact" and "don't hyperextend the knee during support," with no change in results, I am convinced that a team of experts from various areas is needed to effectively design a program which will correct this asymmetry. For example, a review of the high-speed films indicated that this subject had significant pronation of the feet during support. Several weeks before the force platform test, this athlete was examined by a Podiatrist and orthotics were

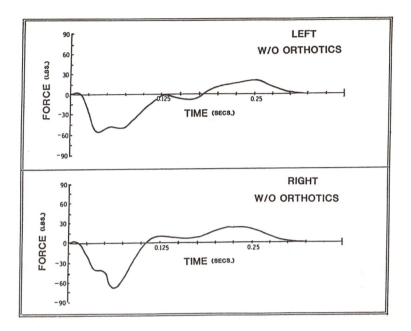

Figure 8.2. Asymmetry between anterior/posterior force patterns for race walking.

prescribed to correct this exaggerated pronation. Thus, in our experi-
mentation, we decided to examine the braking/propulsion curves
with and without orthotics in the shoes. Figure 8.3 illustrates the
frictional force pattern for the right foot with and without orthotics.
With respect to this force component, there didn't seem to be any
large differences in the force patterns between the two conditions.
However, the orthotics did seem to have an affect upon the force
patterns for the left foot. As depicted in Figure 8.4, the orthotics
reduced the duration of the braking phase and increased the time and
level of force for the propulsion period when compared to the non-
orthotic condition. Although these results are very preliminary, they
do indicate the need for biomechanists and podiatrists to relate
together in attempting to solve foot and force transmission problems.

In addition to consulting with medical experts, physiologists
could be included to determine if strength differences might be the
cause of the asymmetry. If movement pattern adjustments are to be
made, perhaps the specialist in motor learning would have some

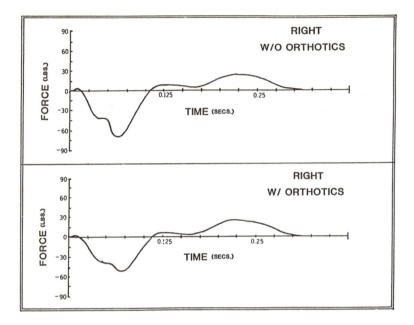

Figure 8.3. Anterior/posterior force patterns: differences in right foot force patterns without and with orthotics.

suggestions as to how these changes might be made. Imagery is a powerful technique that is being used more frequently to improve performance. A psychologist might be able to use the high-speed films from this experiment in conjunction with imagery to effectively develop a smoother leg action. All of these specialists can collectively develop a meaningful program which could correct the problem and result in improved performance.

Cross-Country Skiing

Biomechanical investigations were conducted for the U.S. Nordic Team from 1978 to 1981 to determine the differences in technique between top European and American skiers. A comparative analysis between these two groups indicated that the elite skiers had a stride characterized by a relatively long length and slightly lower stride

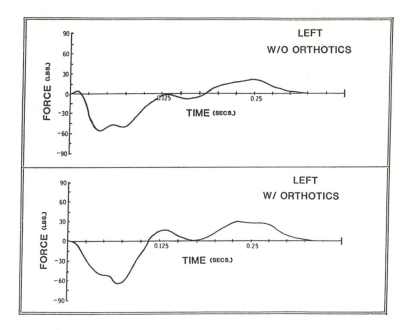

Figure 8.4. Anterior/posterior force patterns: differences in left foot force patterns without and with orthotics.

rate. The major difference between American and top European skiers seems to be stride length. Thus, we concluded that in order to improve our ability to ski fast, U.S. skiers had to increase stride length.

When this finding was implemented into practice, the results were a complete failure. As athletes tried to increase stride length, they developed uncoordinated movement patterns and actually became slower. After considerable thought about this problem, we came to the conclusion that stride length was the wrong teaching concept. Thus, we then focused our efforts upon what were the causes of stride length and increased speed. Based upon this analysis, it was found that elite skiers assume selected balanced body positions and performed movements which allowed for the effective and efficient flow of force to the skis. It was these techniques which produced long strides and allowed the elite skier to travel at a high rate of speed.

Upon reviewing the problem of stride length with one of my colleagues in motor learning, he stated, "Of course that is the wrong teaching concept." If only I had integrated my research with a learning specialist, it probably would have saved me one year of time and eliminated the frustration of a number of coaches and athletes. In addition, the utilization of a psychologist would have been extremely helpful in implementing these results. In conjunction with a physiologist, future work needs to be conducted on the efficiency of skiing and determining how changes in length and rate of striding affect energy output. A strong interdisciplinary approach is needed to solve complex problems such as exist within the sport of cross-country skiing.

SUMMARY

There is no doubt that if the field of sports science is to make further advancements, the various specialized areas must work together in solving the unique and difficult problems of sport. There is some progress being made in this area by several groups, but the examples of true interdisciplinary approaches are few.

Perhaps, however, there is a logical explanation for this lack of integration within the field of sports science. Before someone or a group can relate to other areas, they need the capability of producing results within their own area. It seems that the present status of the specialized areas within sports science have just achieved that level. Each area has solved its technical and methodological procedures and now is applying these experimental protocols in solving theoretical and practical problems. In other words, each individual area has reached maturity and is now searching for other interpretations of results and/or assistance with the implementation of findings. Relative to the development of the entire field, it is probably too early to expect widespread integration among areas. However, if we collectively perceive the need for integration of ideas and knowledge and work toward this goal, there is no doubt that the field of sports science will witness exponential growth and become a truly recognized discipline among the sciences.

REFERENCES

1. Marino, G. W. Multiple regression models of the mechanics of the acceleration phase of ice skating. Unpublished doctoral dissertation, University of Illinois, Urbana-Champaign, IL, 1975.
2. Hatze, H. Computerized optimization of sports motions: An overview of possibilities, methods and recent developments. *Journal of Sports Sciences,* I, 3–12, 1983.

III.
Psychology of Sports

CHAPTER 9

Psychological Aspects of Athletic Performance: An Overview

Jerry R. May

INTRODUCTION

Athletes will benefit if they become knowledgeable regarding the various psychological principles which can enhance their athletic performance. Athletes know that physical training is an extremely important basis for athletic performance. In fact, sports measure ability by a physical performance. Most physical training programs seek to achieve maximum physical conditioning and physical skills levels. The athlete, however, goes beyond physical conditioning and attempts to seek other proper ingredients to assist in the attainment of full potential.

On a given day in competition the difference between one athlete's performance and another's may depend on how well the athlete is prepared mentally. Athletes train hard physically and have specific physical programs, and they also can benefit from developing specific psychological training programs. These programs enhance performance for athletes who regularly utilize them.

The Elite Athlete, edited by N. K. Butts, T. T. Gushiken, and B. Zarins. Copyright © 1985 by Spectrum Publications, Inc.

STRESS

Prior to discussing specific psychological programs which can be developed for athletes and coaches, it is important to understand the concept of stress and its influence upon mental preparation and athletic performance. First, stress cannot and should not be totally avoided. To eliminate it would be to destroy life itself. If no more demands are made upon our body, it is dead. Stress is a vital, creative force that energizes the body. Yet like all powerful forces, it can also throw the body off course. Whatever is done (running a race, competing in a basketball game, taking a test in school, or fighting starvation), demands are made. Although there are good and bad stressors, both make certain demands upon the body requiring adaptation to change from a normal resting state of equilibrium. It is unthinkable that stress can be totally avoided; however, it is important to learn to distinguish which stressors are beneficial and which are detrimental to mental and emotional state and thus effect performance. Everyone must learn to recognize for themselves what is overstress and when the limits of adaptability have been exceeded.

At times athletes feel that they are immune to the influence of stress. This is not true; everyone experiences it. Stress has been defined as "the nonspecific response of the body to any demand upon it" [1]. As the definition indicates, stress is a very general concept. A "nonspecific response" means any physiological or behavioral (performance) response of the body. "Any demand" means any environmental or mental input upon the person. Thus stress includes almost any thought, feeling or event that occurs in one's life.

There are many factors that can cause stress in athletes—some external and others internal. When an athlete is training, many doors may be faced, and the individual must find the key to get through. The doors can be anything from dealing with parents to developing a new maneuver that the athlete has never before carried out.

The external factors are areas that go beyond the control of the athlete, such as boisterous spectators or being over-coached. These are problems that most every athlete experiences and must get used to in the sporting arena. The higher in a sport the athlete goes, the more of these factors seem to develop. The internal factors are areas that the athlete has to learn to control from within, such as lack of sleep, remembering plays, and worrying about mistakes. The athlete must particularly learn to control these factors since we produce them ourselves and they potentially are the easiest to control. When the athlete learns to control internal factors, it is sometimes then easier to limit the effects of external factors. It is when thoughts are difficult to control, feelings too intense, and situations seem overwhelming, that the psychological training program in athletic competition can be most beneficial. Athletes do experience positive and negative stressors.

General Adaptation Syndrome

Three very important stages in the body's response to repeated stress over a long period of time have been identified. When confronted with a stress-producing agent (a stressor), no matter what the particular irritant is, a three-part reaction occurs called the General Adaptation Syndrome [1]. This syndrome consists of (1) the phase of alarm, during which the body is put on alert and summons its defensive forces to combat the stressor; (2) the stage of resistance, where the body maintains and fights against the irritant; and (3) the stage of exhaustion, when unable to resist and attack any longer, the body finally gives into and experiences a breakdown in performance, the onset of disease, or ultimately death. The alarm phase is similar to a time trial or specific event on the day of competition. The body and mind go into action to cope with the stress of the situation and normally do quite well. If, however, the time trials or competitive events continue at close intervals for a longer period of time, the mind and body are kept in the totally ready state, and the responses of the resistance stage are triggered.

Unfortunately, the real situation does not have to be present for the alarm, resistance, and exhaustion sequence to occur, because the mind has the capability to store in memory an event and then worry. The mind and body have the capacity to endure this exposure for a while, but with extensive stress the mind and body break down. Illness and injury rate goes up, and performance level is reduced during this phase. If the stressor continues, the exhaustion stage takes over. This exhaustion is not merely the fatigue experienced after a hard workout; it is serious and can have long-lasting effects on the athlete's mind and body.

Athletes and coaches need to learn the signs of each phase of this stress process for each individual. Noticing one's specific state of mental status and physical health or a marked reduction in performance are excellent clues. For example, during the competitive season, an athlete will experience the alarm phase time and time again. During competition this is the excitement and energy felt just prior to and during competition. If training is too intense and competitions too close, the athlete may begin to experience difficulty in

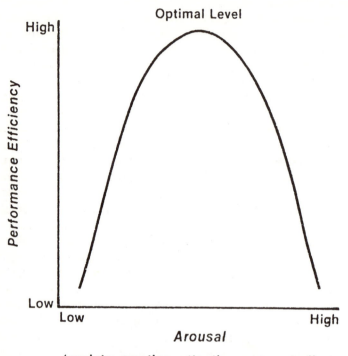

Figure 9.1. Relationship of stress and performance efficiency.

relaxing or will become increasingly cynical about specific aspects of the sport, coach, or fellow athletes. The athlete is now in the resistance phase, and depending on how intense and how long these feelings continue, the athlete may enter the exhaustion phase.

Arousal and Performance

There is a specific relationship between arousal (i.e., anxiety, emotions, attention, concentration, stress, motivation) and athletic performance. Figure 9.1 depicts this relationship. Every athlete needs to understand this relationship and apply it to his own situation. The relationship between arousal and performance reveals that at low levels performance will be inefficient. As arousal increases, perform-ance increases until an optimal level is reached. Further increases in arousal begin to have a detrimental effect and performance diminishes. There is a delicate balance between arousal and performance. For example, the athlete can be about ready to compete, but think of a competitor, a past accident, the crowd of spectators, or something else upsetting. They are immediately placed into the over-aroused state. Every athlete has experienced this phenomenon. What is important is how well the change is detected in the arousal level and what can be done to keep it at an optimal level. Fortunately, arousal levels can be controlled. Once a game, race, or event has begun, everything should be automatic. Psychological preparations can enhance readiness, so athletic performance will be automatic and more natural. It is important to realize that any change in arousal, anxiety, emotions, attention, concentration, stress, and motivation result in the same curvilinear relationship with respect to efficiency of performance. Each athlete needs to know his own optimal level of arousal for peak efficiency. The signs within each athlete for optimal arousal are different. For some athletes it is a feeling of confidence, calm, or peacefulness; for others it is a pleasurable excitement. Some athletes have reported that their minds become almost blank in some sports like skiing or sprinting. At the starting gate, there is a total concentration on the moment and the task at hand. Breathing is usually regular and a desire to perform well is commonly expressed. Again, the characteristics of this optimal level vary from person to person. It is important to distinguish the difference between signs of optimal arousal and overarousal. Overarousal is usually depicted by rapid breathing, muscles feeling tense, anger toward self, and rambling thoughts that are distracting, such as images of the crowds, a competitor, or the weather.

It is important to realize that if the athlete is not doing well but is trying harder, he may actually produce worse results. He may already be trying too hard. Also one can proceed from a low level to a high level of stress within seconds.

Frustration

Another important concept for athletes to understand is the influence of frustration on behavioral actions. Stress or overarousal frequently leads to frustration, which characteristically produces three basic responses in everyone. These responses will negatively influence an athlete's performance. The responses are innate in everyone, but with individuals there is a tendency to use one more than another. The three responses to frustration are (1) anger, (2) fleeing the situation, or (3) freezing. Anger is a primitive emotion that usually indicates that one is out of control. At times it is said that anger is a good motivator; however, this is not true. Anger is an emotional response which is extremely difficult to control. Exceptional performance requires consistency, and since anger is so unpredictable, control is almost impossible, which leads to very inconsistent performances. For example, on a scale of 1 to 10 with 10 being very angry, to say to get angry at five is luck at best. The brain does not control anger directly, and the athlete may be at nine before he knows it. If anger is used toward ourself, competitor, coach, or parent as a motivator, then concentration on the task at hand is distracted. Fleeing a situation means the athlete is not facing up to the event and is trying to avoid or escape or have an excuse. The athlete may refuse to train or try to rationalize getting out of an event. He may flee physically but also can flee mentally and emotionally to avoid or to escape sometimes by concentrating on things other than the task at hand) the event. Finally, freezing is failing to move, feeling tense and locked up, or by feeling caged. This may be experienced as when going down the course the athlete's body feels stiff and inflexible or as when the athlete does not want to leave the room the day of competition. Again, this can be mental or emotional as well as physical. Most people realize that fleeing or freezing a situation will detrimentally effect performance. Again, when any one of these responses occur due to frustration, performance will become inconsistent and out of control.

Coaches need to be aware that they are also susceptible to stress, and its influence on their performance is effected in ways very similar to athletes. To be a good coach, one needs to be aware of these principles as they apply to oneself as well as the athlete.

STRESS MANAGEMENT OR COPING STRATEGIES FOR PERFORMANCE ENHANCEMENT

There is a five-step process that athletes need to undergo as they develop their own personal stress management program. These five steps are

1. Identify the sources of increased levels of stress and examine how stress is affecting thoughts, feeling, and behavior (performance).
2. Decide on specific coping strategies.

3. Develop an individual action plan for coping.
4. Practice specific coping and relaxing skills.
5. Review the effectiveness of these skills and redesign as needed.

The next sections of this chapter deal with the development of a personal stress management program designed to improve athletic performance.

Identification of Stress

First it is important to identify how stress is experienced (thoughts, feelings, and performance) and what the stressors are in one's life. Table 9.1 depicts some general signs and symptoms of stress.

These signs and symptoms are only a few of the indicators of stress in our lives. Everyone has experienced one or more of these signs at times. It is the number, frequency, duration, and intensity of these factors that indicate the seriousness of the stress. It is important to identify the stressors; if indicated, the athlete should do something to reduce or to eliminate them.

One of the first steps in coping with stress is to acknowledge its influence. Next try to reduce it. There is no such thing as a quick fix. Learning to cope effectively takes time, effort, and practice. Look carefully at your life, at how you live, and at what you want to do. Slowing down your life, trying not to be everything to everybody, learning how to relax, getting plenty of sleep, and setting time aside for fun are all basic principles of having an enjoyable life and enhancing performance. This does not mean to be lazy. Training and work are important. Allowing time to laugh and spend time with family and friends and not just concentrating on athletics is, however, a necessary ingredient to success.

If you find yourself experiencing stress and are heading for (or have arrived at) the exhaustion phase, it is helpful to slow down the pace of your life, refocus your goals, and reshape your expectations. Six basic guidelines to help counteract the negative effects of stress are

1. Forgive yourself (with no strings attached).
2. Forgive others.
3. Don't compare yourself to others.
4. See your good side.

Table 9.1. A Checklist of Warning Signs of Negative Stress

Physical Signs

[ ] Fatigue
[ ] Pounding of the heart
[ ] Dryness of the throat or mouth
[ ] Insomnia, an inability to fall asleep, stay asleep, or early awakenings
[ ] Frequent or lingering colds
[ ] Trembling and nervous ticks
[ ] Grinding of the teeth
[ ] Increase or decrease in appetite
[ ] Increased sweating
[ ] Frequent need to urinate
[ ] Diarrhea
[ ] Indigestion, queaziness in the stomach
[ ] Vomiting
[ ] Pain in neck or lower back
[ ] Increased premenstrual tension
[ ] Missed menstrual cycle
[ ] Headache
[ ] Weakness
[ ] Dizziness
[ ] Weight gain or loss
[ ] Shortness of breath
[ ] Stuttering or other speech difficulties
[ ] Increased pitch in voice
[ ] Nervous laughter

Emotional Signs

[ ] General irritability
[ ] Hyperexcitability
[ ] Depression
[ ] Boredom
[ ] Restlessness
[ ] Stagnation
[ ] Overpowering urge to cry, run, or hide
[ ] Difficulty relaxing
[ ] Need to generate excitement over and over
[ ] Feeling people don't appreciate you, feeling used
[ ] Inability to laugh at yourself
[ ] Increased feeling of expression of anger or being cynical
[ ] Inability to concentrate, the flight of thoughts
[ ] Disenchantment
[ ] Feeling of unreality
[ ] Feeling life is not much fun
[ ] Not enjoying your sport

Emotional Signs (Continued)

[　] Desire to quit the team
[　] Mind going blank
[　] Feeling afraid
[　] "Free floating anxiety," that is to say we are afraid of something but we don't know exactly what it is
[　] Feel under pressure to always succeed
[　] Hyperalertness, a feeling of being "keyed up"
[　] Automatic expression of negative feelings
[　] Disappointed in yourself or others
[　] Increased rationalization
[　] Feeling indispensable
[　] Obsessed
[　] Unable to enjoy or compliment colleagues' successes
[　] Fault finding
[　] Nightmares

Behavioral Signs

[　] Tendency to overtrain
[　] Difficulty training
[　] Decrease in athletic performance
[　] Increased use of alcohol
[　] Increased use of nonprescribed drugs
[　] Increased use of various medications, such as tranquilizers or amphetamines
[　] Increased use of tobacco
[　] Less time for recreation
[　] Less time for intimacy with people around you
[　] Less vacation time
[　] Overworked, but can't say no to more work without feeling guilty
[　] Hypermotility, which is the increased tendency to move about without any reason
[　] Inability to take a physically relaxed attitude, such as sitting quiet in a chair or lying on a sofa
[　] Feeling that sex is more trouble than its worth
[　] Speaking up less and less at gatherings, and then only speaking negatively
[　] Difficulty setting goals
[　] A tendency to be easily startled by small sounds
[　] Finding yourself further behind at the end of each day
[　] Forgetting deadlines, appointments, etc.
[　] Accident proneness (under great stress whether it is positive or negative, one is more likely to have accidents while at work, driving a car, or during athletic events)
[　] Making a foolish mistake
[　] Poor workout
[　] Blame equipment for poor performance

5. See the good in others.
6. Be positive about today (don't dwell in the past or future).

Most of the following training programs are used to enhance performance skills, and many of them deal with how to appropriately control tension and stress levels. Each of these programs has been found useful. Start with one or two programs which are personally suitable or fit a particular time or situation. Do not try to learn too many at one time or overload will occur and the effects of the techniques will not reach full potential. All these programs require that the athlete practice these techniques as regularly as any physical training exercises would be practiced. *Psychological exercise, like physical exercise, does not work if it is not used on a continuous basis.* If these techniques are used on a regular basis, they will be very effective in the prevention and control of negative stress.

Relaxation Training Program

The relaxation training program can be one of the most beneficial psychological techniques to keep the athlete at an optimal level of performance. These exercises should be conducted on a daily basis for ten to fifteen minutes, and then if the athlete feels situationally tense just prior to competition, the sensation of relaxation can be recalled mentally within just a few seconds. In practicing the relaxation technique, it is first important to pay attention to the environment. The relaxation training should take place in a quiet surrounding that is comfortable and will facilitate maximal concentration. The technique outlined is based upon a method described by Bernstein and Borkovec [2]. The procedure allows the athlete to deeply relax various muscle groups of the body.

There is a specific sequence which needs to be followed:

1. Attention should focus on the specific muscle group.
2. A specific muscle group is to be tensed.
3. Tension is maintained for a period of 5 to 7 seconds (this duration is shorter in the case of the feet).
4. The muscle group tension is then released.
5. Attention should be maintained on the muscle group as it relaxes for an additional 20 to 30 seconds.

Remember that the goal of progressive relaxation training is to help learn to reduce the muscle tension in the body far below levels normally achieved. The procedure produces relaxation in sixteen specific muscle groups.

While you are relaxing, it is important to concentrate on breathing. Breathe normally while relaxing but during each exhale or breath out, think of pushing the tension out of the body. The muscles of the body normally contract or get tense with breathing in and release and relax with breathing out. Synchronizing this breathing out as you are also concentrating on relaxing the muscles can enhance the effect.

Step 1:   Let's begin with the dominant hand and forearm (for most people this will be the right hand and right lower arm). Tense the right hand and right lower arm by making a tight fist. Now you should be able to feel the tension in the hand over the knuckles and up into the lower arm. Focus attention on that muscle group and maintain that tension for five to seven seconds. Release that tension and maintain focus on the relaxation feelings for approximately 20 to 30 seconds. A tingling or warming sensation may be felt. Between the tension and release, contrast the relaxation state with the tension state and "zero in" on the relaxation state.

Step 2:   Now move to the muscles of the upper arm. Tense these muscles by pushing the elbows down against the floor if lying down or the arm of a chair if sitting. A feeling of tension should occur in the upper arm without involving the muscles in the lower arm and hand. Once the tension is developed, stop and allow those muscles to relax; concentrate on the relaxation.

Step 3:   Tense the nondominant hand and forearm by clenching the fist. Hold, then relax.

Step 4:   Now tense the nondominant upper arm by pushing down with the arm or elbow on the floor or the arm of a chair. Hold the tension, let it release and relax. After relaxing the arms and hands, relax the muscles of the face. This will be divided into three muscle groups: The first muscle is in the forehead (the upper part of the face), then the muscles of the central part of the face (the upper part of the cheeks and the nose), and finally the lower part of the face (the jaws and lower part of the cheeks).

Step 5:   Tense the muscles of the forehead by lifting up the eyebrows just as high as possible and getting the tension in the forehead and up into the scalp region. Hold that tension and then let it relax and zero in on the sensations of relaxation.

Step 6:   Now move down to the muscles in the central part of the face. In order to tense these muscles, squint the eyes very tightly and at the same time wrinkle up the nose and get tension through the central part of the face. The tension should be in the upper part of the cheeks and through the eye region. Hold this tension, then let it relax for 20 to 30 seconds concentrating again on the sensations experienced.

Step 7:   Next tense the muscles in the lower part of the face. To do this, bite the teeth together and pull the corners of the mouth back. This is like a smile with the teeth clamped together. Tension will be felt all through the lower part of the face and jaw. Once the tension is developed, let the muscles relax and again experience those sensations.

Step 8:   Now pull the chin downward to the chest and at the same time try to prevent it from actually touching the chest. This will counterpose muscles in the front part of the neck against those in the back of the neck. A little bit of shaking and trembling may be felt in these muscles as they are tensed. Hold them tight for a few seconds, then let them release. Immediately concentrate on the sensations of relaxation by release of those tense muscles.

Step 9:   Now move to the muscles of the chest, the shoulders, and upper back. A few of these muscles will be combined here. Tense these muscles by taking a deep breath, holding, and at the same time pulling the shoulder blades together, that is, pull the shoulder blades back and try to make the shoulder blades touch. Significant tension will be felt in the chest, shoulders, and the upper back. Hold that tension, let it release, and notice the sensations of relaxation; concentrate only on the feelings of relaxation.

Step 10:   Now move to the muscles of abdomen. In order to make those tight, tense up the abdomen or stomach muscles as though you were going to hit yourself in the stomach. A good deal of tension and tightness will be felt in the stomach. As soon as this tension is developed, let it relax. Remember to synchronize breathing as relaxing is attempted; attempt to let the relaxation go further and further. Each time you breathe out, more and more tension is being released from the body. After relaxing the muscles of the stomach, you will now move on to the muscles of the legs and feet.

Step 11: Tense the muscles of the right-upper leg by lifting the leg straight out and noticing the tension in the muscles above the knee. Hold that tension, let it release, and concentrate on the relaxation.

Step 12: Now move to the muscles of the right calf and right-lower leg. With the foot and leg resting level on the ground with support, pull the toes upward toward the head. Tension will now be felt through the calf area. Hold that tension and then let it release and relax.

Step 13: Now move to the muscles of the right foot. Point the toes and turn the foot inward at the same time curling the toes; don't tense these muscles very hard, just enough to feel tightness under the arch and the ball of the foot. Notice the tension, let it release, and concentrate on the relaxation sensations. Again these may be warmth and tingling. Now move to the muscles of the upper leg, lower leg and foot.

Step 14: Just as with the right leg, tense the upper-left leg by holding the leg out and up from the ground. Notice that tension, let the leg drop, and concentrate on the relaxation.

Step 15: Now with the left leg or nondominant calf, tense the muscles by pulling the toes upward toward the head. Note the tension, then let the muscles relax.

Step 16: Now with the nondominant foot, point the toes outward, turn the foot inward, and curl the toes, noticing the tension. Again don't tense the muscles very hard. Let the muscles relax.

After having gone through the sixteen muscle groups, attempt to concentrate specifically on each of the sixteen muscle groups. Synchronize breathing with the deepening of relaxation. Attempting to recall these states of relaxation in each muscle group just after practicing the technique will enhance the chances of later being able to recall the relaxation procedure when there is an athletic situation where tension is felt but all the physical maneuvers cannot be completed.

Remember, these exercises should be practiced ten to fifteen minutes each day. A coach or a friend may verbally give these instructions as the technique is learned. Coaches can give these relaxation exercise instructions to a group of athletes. It may be beneficial to make an audiotape of the sixteen steps for listening to the tape while learning and practicing the technique. Playing some calming, meditative music before, during, and after the instructions on tape can make the experience more pleasant.

Recall these sensations prior to or during excessive stress producing times. The morning of an event or just prior to competition, these sensations of relaxation can be recalled. Some sports allow the opportunity of utilizing this procedure during the athletic activity when tension levels are becoming too great. Simply close the eyes and mentally go through each muscle group, bringing back the sensations of warm tingling or heaviness. This can be done in just a few moments, and if the techniques are practiced on a daily basis, they will have a very positive effect. This will help keep the arousal level to its optimum.

GOALS AND INCENTIVES

In helping to stay focused and motivated and to cope with stress, it is important to know one's goals and to understand why one becomes involved in a sport.

Goals

Each individual at some level needs to be aware of goals. It is best to write them down, but this is not necessary for everyone. The main thing to remember about goals is that realistic ones must be set. Goals need to be understood on three levels. There are short-term goals, intermediate goals, and long-term goals. An example of a long-term goal may be making the Olympic Team or even winning a medal. The amount of time spent thinking about long-term goals should be minimal. Intermediate goals could be doing well during a particular time in the season, performing at a particular level during a specific competition, or making a desired level of national team

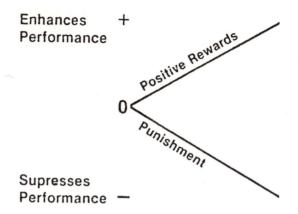

Figure 9.2. Effects of positive reward and punishment on performance.

involvement. Again these intermediate goals help keep thoughts in perspective but need not be reviewed on a daily basis.

Short-term goals deal with specific training programs and their component parts; for example, building up of physical endurance capacity and psychological training. Short-term goals also assist enhancement of a specific skill or work on a specific problem area for the day or week. Athletic performance is improved by paying attention to the basic physical and psychological principles underlying the sport. This is where most of the effort should be most of the time.

It is important to remember that goals are usually some arbitrary means of setting specific expectations. Goals have to be continually revised and made realistic, given the situation. Too often people tend to be rigid about goal setting. Goals can be and probably should be changed periodically.

A very significant principle in the psychology of sport is to make sure that more positive rewards for being involved are received than negative feedback. If long-term, intermediate, or short-term goals are set too high, we will continuously feel upset and negative. Reinforcing oneself in such a negative way is called punishment. Figure 9.2 demonstrates the effect of positive reward and punishment upon behavior.

A positive reward, such as a feeling of a job well done is important and will enhance performance and increase the chances of getting better at the desired activity. The plus signs (+) on this figure show how performance increases if there are positive rewards.

Likewise, it is known that punishment suppresses or reduces the frequency of a given behavior. Therefore, it is appropriate at times to have a negative thought or to receive some negative feedback about something that we do not want to do any more. However, if there is too much punishment, very serious effects can occur. The serious side effects of punishment are decreased self-esteem, increased self-doubt, and decreased emotional stability. People who have been too critical of themselves or have received too much criticism will experience more anger, anxiety, and depression than those who do not. They also will not perform as well. The side effects of positive reward are all beneficial. They include increased self-esteem, increased performance level, and a feeling of well-being. Even if one is not doing something well, rather than merely pointing out the error or being negative for making the error, it is better to point out the correction or even attempt to "zero in" and practice that correction. The desired behavior is thus being performed, and there is a greater probability of positive reward. This is a concept that coaches also need to learn. Pointing out the error may only punish the athlete; whereas if the athlete is given positive feedback or is made aware of the correction, he can practice that correction, feel better, and enhance performance. Again, a delicate balance is indicated. Examine what can be done!

Incentives

Along with goals, positive reward and punishment is the concept of incentives. What is it that makes the athlete work so long and hard, practice for hours, develop self-discipline, and endure loneliness? What makes this sacrifice worthwhile? Each athlete must know for himself what the incentives are. Again, long-term incentives may be recognition, winning a gold medal, being a team member on an U.S. Olympic Team. These incentives are sometimes difficult to reach and to experience. It is best to have incentives which can be felt on a more frequent basis. Incentives listed by elite athletes are frequently that their sport is fun, they enjoy being physically fit, they enjoy competition, and they enjoy the sense of self-improvement. Others have related that they enjoy the relationship with the coach or being together with the team. They also feel parental and peer support in what they are doing, and of course, most enjoy performing well and ultimately winning.

Most world-class athletes have developed what are called "internal" as well as "external" rewards or incentives. This helps them to keep going. The external goals of recognition and possibly money are important, but to excel, an athlete must develop internal incentives of self-satisfaction, fun, etc. For it is the athlete that understands himself, receives satisfaction from within, and basically likes himself, who will be the consistent achiever.

Most sports are a measurable activity which makes it one of the few areas in life where a person can be judged the best in the world. Yet surprisingly, wanting to be a gold-medal winner or world-record holder is not a good motivator if it is the major or single motivator. The athlete who says, "I'm going to break a world record no matter what" is generally focusing so hard on glory in the future that he may lose sight of the present and the athlete may not properly train for or compete in the intermediate events.

To succeed, athletes and their coaches need to be realistic and know their incentives, motivations, and goals. It is rare that the top athlete goes all out simply to be "number one" or only to "win." Rather these top athletes attempt to excel in their field: "I am going to do the best job I can!" With this striving for excellence, they end up winning a variety of world-class honors.

COGNITIVE RESTRUCTURING: POSITIVE THINKING

Cognitive restructuring is a technique which can help the athlete to learn to think more positively and reduce the number of derogatory or overqualifying statements relating to performance. Having doubts is normal, but when they become pervasive, they interfere with performance. Always qualifying what is said or thought (for example, "I am a good golfer, but I tend to slice") usually has the same effect as derogatory statements. Cognitive restructuring is a means of learning to cope with the mental sentences that are repeatedly said to ourselves which can effect performance adversely. Examples of the negative mental sentences are

"I wonder if I practiced hard enough."
"I know that so and so is better than I am."
"I just can't seem to make the free throws."
"I do not jump well when it's raining."
"My equipment is probably not as good as my competitors."

In an athlete's daily life, a considerable amount of time is spent thinking. Unfortunately, much of this thinking is negative. This relates back to the concept of positive rewards in Figure 9.2. If there are more negative thoughts going on than positive ones, this will detrimentally affect performance and result in the side effects of low self-esteem and depression.

The four steps of the restructuring technique are

Step 1: Identify statements that you are saying to yourself.
Step 2: Change the statements to more realistic and positive ones.
Step 3: Practice each positive statement.
Step 4: Evaluate and assess whether more positive statements than negative statements are being said.

A specific example of cognitive restructuring in alpine skiing would be when the athlete is standing on top of the hill and notices that his competitor has just had a very fast time. Many athletes might say to themselves or out loud, "I'm fearful that I cannot do as well now that he has had such a good time." The cognitive restructuring statement would be, "Great! He's just had a good run. The course must be in great shape. Now I can really go for it." Another example would be, on a windy day after watching a competitor have difficulty being accurate during an archery competition, one might say, "Oh, if they can't shoot in the wind, how can I." Another example of restructuring into a more positive vein and one that can be controlled would be, "It is windy. I have practiced shooting in the wind, and I know how to compensate for it."

It is known that people, although they may say something good about themselves, tend to qualify the good with a negative. An example of this would be, "I had a good first run, *but* my skis didn't feel right," or "I can keep a good line, *but* I have difficulty with left turns." Saying this negative qualification essentially negates the feeling about doing something well. It is necessary to separate what is done well from what is not done as well. Try to balance in the positive direction thoughts about what is done well versus what is not done as well.

Affirmations

The concept of affirmations is a variant of cognitive restructuring. Affirmations are realistic and positive sentences said to oneself. The affirmation may be a little exaggerated to make the point. An example of an affirmation statement would be, "I enjoy tennis," or

"I like myself," or "I enjoy other people." Saying these statements four or five times a day can help one feel more confident with oneself and less negative toward others or things that may be done.

Four or five affirmations specific to oneself can be developed and then repeated four or five times in a row at a given situation. Specific affirmations regarding practice or competition can be made up. Affirmation for practice would be, "I enjoy my training and I am doing well." An affirmation for competition may be, "I peak when I'm in competition," or "I find lots of satisfaction from playing football."

Sometimes distractions occur in thinking negatively about fellow athletes and competitors. An affirmation which helps reduce those negative thoughts and stress level is, "I have warm positive regard for all people at all times." Although this may sound exaggerated, the repetition of this statement will reduce tension levels in stressful interpersonal situations. It is important that these statements are tried and practiced, saying them four or five times in succession when there is no stressful situation, and then utilizing them when the stressful situation is present. The positive effect will be surprising!

Visual Imagery Training

Imagery training is the ability to evoke a vivid image like a real picture in the mind. We all have the potential for producing pictures in our minds, but like anything else it must be practiced. When attempting to produce a visual image, the more specific one can make that image, the more vivid the image will be. If possible, it is best to use as many of the five senses as possible while producing an image. For example, you will visualize but at the same time bring in the sense of touch, smell, hearing, and taste if it is applicable. Attempt to feel the experience as much as possible. In skiing, try to visualize the ski hill; feel the coolness of the day, the heat of the sun, and smell the fresh air; see the beauty of the trees; and also physically feel the ski on the snow. Visual imagery is the first step before mental rehearsal, and being able to specifically visualize the situation as totally as possible is very important.

Mental Rehearsal

Mental rehearsal simply involves practicing as a visual image an athletic technique, procedure, or event in one's mind. Initially this can be done step by step. As the athlete becomes proficient in this skill, one can slow down or speed up the rehearsal, until one is in total synchronization with the flow of the body, mind, and action. Since mental rehearsal can be arousing, it is best not to do this at bedtime but at some other time during the day. It's helpful if mental rehearsal is practiced initially in a quiet and calm place. It can be used alone or in conjunction with the relaxation techniques. A specific event like ice skating can be recalled and gone over in detail. Visualize yourself on the ice, moving with grace, power, ease, and coordination. One of the unique abilities of the mind is that the situations can be changed as seen fit. If a skier, you may want to see yourself in practice, racing on a beautiful, sunny day where the snow conditions are perfect, or you may want to practice doing well on the day when it's snowy, windy, and conditions are not really optimal. In addition, specific techniques or specific parts of a race hill can be practiced in the mind. Frequently a videotape of a good role model who skis similarly to yourself, or a videotape of yourself skiing, can act as good stimulus material for producing visual imagery and mental rehearsal. As you are practicing, you may even see yourself making an error. The nice thing about mental rehearsal is that it can be stopped, then the corrective maneuver can be practiced without having undergone the physical ramifications (a crash, fall, or injury) of that error.

Coupling the relaxation exercises with mental rehearsal helps reduce the stress, while visualizing competition. Then when in competition, relaxation is already associated with carrying out that event. Athletes have found this technique to be very helpful in controlling stress levels and maximizing performance.

Parents, coaches, and fellow athletes can serve as guides or facilitators in mental rehearsal. They can help the athlete identify what needs to be known and help direct the training. This should not be done in an authoritative dictator's style if the athlete is to succeed. Frequently, having someone say or suggest the particular mental rehearsal activity while the athlete is relaxing is helpful.

With mental rehearsal attempt to make the activity as real as possible. Some people have found that writing out the activity to be rehearsed is helpful in the initial stages. Some athletes find initially that it is easier to imagine themselves watching as a spectator as they are practicing the particular event. Then later on, when one can really feel oneself in the mental rehearsal, it will probably have a greater effect.

Stop-Thinking Technique

The stop-thinking technique is a procedure for eliminating unwanted and distracting thoughts. All too often during the day of competition, or on the prior evening (while trying to fall asleep), one finds oneself with a mind full of negative and worrisome thoughts. Most people say that they would like to stop these thoughts because they detrimentally affect performance or keep them from falling asleep. Unfortunately, simply saying that you do not want a thought does not get rid of it. In fact, by saying that a thought is not wanted means the thought has just been repeated again and the whole vicious cycle is continued. There is a very straightforward procedure for eliminating unwanted thoughts. This procedure can be very effective but should not be utilized to deny or to eliminate thoughts when there is an important issue to be confronted. It is much better to work out the problem rather than simply to eliminate concern. There are, however, specific times when trying to work something out is not appropriate. This is true when trying to fall asleep or at an event just prior to competition. It is also useful during those times between events in sports that have more than one event. There are three basic steps to this procedure:

Step 1: Simply to yourself or out loud say, "Stop!"
Step 2: As soon as you have said, "Stop," produce a very positive and calming image in your mind.
Step 3: Go do something else for just a few moments, if possible.

Utilizing this technique is much more than simply saying, "Stop!" to oneself. Saying "stop" interferes with the thought process. With Step 2, a very positive image is produced in the mind that is calming and has the same effect as a positive reward. Remember, you are trying to stop a thought. When this cessation of a thought is positively rewarded, the chances that the thought will not come back is increased. Finally, if possible, do something else. This creates activity and helps break thought patterns. Stop thinking is a simple conditioning technique and should be utilized when there is a reoccurring disruptive thought. It must be practiced each time the thought comes up so that the thinking of that thought will be conditioned out. An example could be that on the day of the competition there is a tendency to think too much about competitors. As the thought evolves in the mind, simply say, "Stop!" Produce an image of a calm and peaceful situation, and do something else for a few seconds or minutes. One of the things that makes the technique so effective is that it deals on a cognitive or thinking level, an affective or emotional level, and a behavioral or doing level. The first two steps of this program are the most important. There will be times that doing something else is impossible because the situation will not allow it, but the two mental steps, stop and positive image, can be done in the mind. Also if combined with relaxation, the effect can even be greater.

It is suggested that a list is made of four or five positive, calming experiences. These should be practiced through visual imagery so that when they are needed, they can be recalled immediately. It is extremely important that Step 2 follows the "stop" immediately. An example of a positive, calming thought or image might be lying on a beach feeling the sun come down, smelling the freshness of the air, and the wonderful state of relaxation.

Active Rest

Although not a specific technique per se, a very important factor in an overall training program is knowing how and when to take breaks. Active rest refers to these breaks. Specifically, active rest refers to the fact that the athlete still participates in some physical activity but not with the goal of preparing for competition. Active rest is an important concept during the training phases as well as the competition phases of a sport. Knowing when to take breaks throughout the day or for a day during the week, or for several weeks during the off season is important. One of the most detrimental influences on athletic performance is overtraining. Active rest is not to be used as an excuse to be lazy. One should continue some type of physical training to stay fit. However, the intensity that is frequently required of a very competitive training or competitive schedule needs to be reduced at times. Often, the athlete is not aware of this need, and a coach, a peer, or a parent can give cues as to when to follow this active rest procedure. Active rest is an important coping strategy for dealing with stress, exhaustion phase symptoms, and burnout. The signs of negative stress listed in Table 9.1 provide an indication when to use active rest. Active rest should be a systematic part of everyone's psychological program because of its powerful influence on preventing the negative signs of stress, exhaustion, and burnout. Make the time during rest productive with a main goal of enjoying the activity.

Communications

Although it has been attempted to keep this chapter specific to individual techniques, it is difficult to talk about the psychology of sport without talking about communications skills. This section should probably be the beginning of a chapter rather than the end. The ways that athletes communicate to their peers, coaches, and parents have a tremendous effect upon tension levels of all involved. Remember that positive communication increases positive self-esteem, not only within ourselves but within others around us. As relationship tension develops, there is no doubt that the quality of coaching and performance diminishes. This is not only true in athletics, but in other areas of our lives as relationships are developed. There are six principles that will increase relationship tension that need to be remembered:

1. *Judging*: Judging another person by what is said or by the tone of voice will put that other person on the defensive, e.g., "You are not as good an athlete as I." Giving a response which indicates right or wrong continually is a very judgmental style, e.g., "You made that hand-off entirely wrong."

2. *Acting superior*: Acting superior evolves out of judging and acting as though we know what is right, e.g., "Listen, you know I have more experience than you, so just listen." Almost always there is more than one way to look at a particular situation. Acting superior is a very defensive type of response and often indicates insecurity.

3. *Control*: Trying to control someone else is generally going to lead to trouble, and one will find it is very unsuccessful, e.g., "I told you what to do this morning. Why didn't you do it?" It is important to make an attempt to listen to rather than try to control individuals.

4. *Strategy*: If you deal with people as if they are just pawns in an overall plan and as if the situation is just a contest in winning, then individuals are going to feel tense and the relationship is going to deteriorate; e.g., a coach may be pushing an athlete so the coach can get recognition.

5. *Self-centered*: Acting as if there is no concern about other peoples' problems, e.g., "If you think you have problems, you should see what kind of a day I have had."

6. *Opinionated*: Acting like you have all the answers and as if you are the teacher and other people need to be taught is a

direct line to increasing relationship tension, e.g., "The coach doesn't know how I pitch; I am the only one who knows." Be aware of how you are coming across. Ask others what they think of your behavior and attitude.

There are several useful ways to defuse or reduce relationship tension and encourage nondefensive behavior in those with whom an attempt to communicate is made. Remember that a positive communication will increase self-esteem, whereas negative communication will result in bad feelings. In attempting to defuse relationship tension it is helpful to

1. *Try to understand*: Ask questions such as, "Can you tell me more about it?" Gathering more information will help both parties. Watch asking, "Why do you feel that way?" or "Why do you do this?" Questions that begin with "why" will tend to put people on the defensive and make them feel that they must account for their behavior. Making statements such as, "I would like to understand this further," or "What do you think about this?" will lead to a reduction in relationship tension.

2. *Equality*: It is important to avoid acting superior. Place yourself at an equal level with the person to whom you are communicating.

3. *Problem solve*: Problem solving versus trying to control will assist in developing better relationships. Again, do not try to problem solve other peoples' concerns too early. It is important first to try to get information and to understand and then make sure you are acting on an equal basis before problem solving should occur. Also it is important to have the individual who has the problem first to look at possible solutions. Quite often an individual can come up with his or her own ideas if there is a facilitator. All too often, an individual will jump in too quickly in solving someone else's problems but they are not at a point where they can hear, and failure will result. It is best if people come up with their own solutions.

4. *Flexibility*: Again, strategy can be a very detrimental concept. Do not come up with too rigid a plan. Remain flexible and see what other possibilities exist.

5. *Sharing the other person's feelings*: The opposite of being self-centered is trying to understand and empathize with the

other individual's feelings. An example of this would be, "I hear you're angry, and I would be too" rather than simply stating your feelings on the matter: "You think you're angry; I am really mad!"

6. *Open minded*: Again try not to show yourself as being overly opinionated. Demonstrate that you would really like to hear what is going on.

Many of the six points which increase relationship tension and the six points which decrease relationship tension build on one another and overlap. Since it is known that tension can detrimentally affect performance, and that relationships are central to an individual's satisfaction, it will be to our benefit to keep some of these principles in mind. There is much more to communication styles and techniques; however, understanding some basics to relationship development is a start.

CONCLUSION

Many of the psychological techniques discussed have been proven to enhance performance and enable an individual to be calmer and more self-assured. These are simple techniques, and the psychology of sport is actually much more complex. At times it is important to consult a psychologist regarding some of the fine tuning of these various techniques. Unfortunately, sports psychology has individuals involved who are not trained as psychologists. If you seek to consult a psychologist on further issues to enhance performance or deal with the stresses of competition, I suggest that you follow the criteria set down by the U.S. Olympic Sports Psychology Committee. Briefly, the guidelines specify three areas in which psychologists may have expertise: (1) clinical, (2) educational, and (3) research. If one feels that there are some problems in controlling emotions, undergoing considerable crises, or having difficulty in one's own personal growth, a clinical psychologist should be contacted. For specific skill development on some of the aforementioned techniques of relaxation, concentration, and visualization, a psychologist who also meets the criteria as an educational psychologist should be contacted. Usually clinical psychologists also have this ability. Educational psychologist are not trained to get involved in the functions of a clinical psychologist. The research category does not have immediate impact on the athlete, but participation in research enables psychologists to better understand what helps the athlete. For a more detailed understanding of the U.S. Olympic Committee's recommendations for criteria for psychologists involved in sport, one should review the article by Waitley, May, and Martens [3].

REFERENCES

1. Selye, H. *The stress of life*. New York: McGraw-Hill, 1956.
2. Bernstein, D. A., and Borkovec, T. D. *Progressive relaxation training: A manual for the helping professions*. Champagne, ILL: Research Press, 1973.
3. Waitley, D. E., May, J. R., and Martens, R. Sports psychology and the elite athlete. *Clinics in Sports Medicine*, 2(1), 87-100, 1983.

CHAPTER **10**

Cognitive Skills and Strategies for Maximizing Performance

Dorothy V. Harris

The difference between the best performance and the worst performance of any athlete, or the difference between an athlete's practice and performance in competition, can generally be explained by the fluctuation and variation of the mental aspects of performance. Athletes simply do not lose and gain skill and stamina over the course of a single game in a manner that explains their fluctuation in performance! In the final analysis, with all other things being equal, it is not the physical skill that the athlete takes to the competition that counts; it is the psychological skill that will determine the degree of success in competition. Most athletes are accustomed to practicing physical skills and strategies to improve their performance; few are coached to practice cognitive or mental skills on a regular basis. These skills are just as essential to performance as the physical ones and must be taught and practiced on a regular basis. Inconsistency in performance is explained by lack of mental control.

Lengthy discussions have taken place with regard to what percentage of performance is psychological in competition. In the final analysis, it really does not matter, because it is the critical percent!

The Elite Athlete, edited by N. K. Butts, T. T. Gushiken, and B. Zarins. Copyright © 1985 by Spectrum Publications, Inc.

The observable differences in performance among athletes of relatively equal athletic skill appear to be determined by the athletes' ability to cope with the perceived stress of the competitive situation. Un certainty or worry about the competitive event procedures anxiety that is manifested in both somatic and cognitive ways. Without regulation of this arousal, anxiety can increase to the point that it disrupts cognitive and physical control in such a way that it interferes with performance.

Knowledge of the mental effects on competitive sport is at about the same stage as that known about the physical effects 25 years ago. The approach to training was to play hard at the sport to prepare for competition. There were no special weight training programs, special diets, stretching, or special programs for preparation other than spending a lot of time scrimmaging. The basic idea was that one got better at what they were doing by doing it. The emphasis on pre-peration has always been focused on the physical aspects of performance. Rarely do coaches discuss any psychological preparation; they assume that the athletes can take care of that on their own. In fact, those who do not learn to cope to some degree to ensure fairly consistent performance over time get eliminated from the system. Coaches do not like athletes that they cannot depend on under pressure. Many athletes with all the necessary physical attributes have been cut from teams when they were identified as "chokers." Other athletes have consistently been good "practice" performers but have never been able to equal those performances in competition. Yet another group of athletes may display wildly fluctuating abilities, playing superbly on occasion and poorly at other times. The explanation is always, "the ability is there; he/she just cannot get it together."

Coaches generally attempt to develop tough mindedness in athletes by ranting and raving, insulting, degrading and berating in an attempt to motivate the athlete to better performance by provoking him or her. A few athletes will respond according to the coach's wishes just to prove a point; however, most will never perform to their maximal potential. Athletes who have their anxiety roused by practice and competitive situations generally experience some decrements in their performance. Most coaches do not realize that many of their coaching strategies are counterproductive for the majority of athletes. There are several approaches that reach the same desired end, that being to maximize the athlete's potential.

PHYSICAL PRACTICE IS NOT ENOUGH

Practicing diligently throughout the season, getting rousing pep talks before competition, playing hard, and hoping to win do not provide proper preparation for maximizing one's athletic potential. Based on what we know at this point in time, coaches who fail to systematically prepare their athletes mentally are not doing an adequate job of coaching. Invariably, when athletes fail to meet the coach's expectations in competition, the explanations for lack of success are generally attributed to the mental aspects of the performance. How many times do you hear or read: "We weren't mentally prepared," "We lost our poise," "We lost our momentum," "We lost our concentration?" Athletes deserve the best preparation they can get for all the time and effort they put forth to improve their performance.

Performance is the result of stamina, strength, flexibility, coordination, game skill, and knowledge. However, if the mind is occupied with distracting thoughts or is continuously interrupted with thoughts that interfere with concentration, it cannot coordinate all the necessary factors that contribute to maximal performance. If the mind is not free to "let it happen," the other components of performance will not reach their full potential either. Despite the fact that each athlete faces similar competitive conditions in a single game, each brings to that situation a different personality and a different set of previous experiences. Even with extensive experience in competitive situations, many athletes continue to deny themselves the full benefit of their talents by allowing psychological states that are not conducive to consistently good performance interfere with execution. "Good ol' Charlie Brown" is a perfect example of poor mental preparation and of allowing distracting thoughts to interfere with his performance. He is forever talking himself out of a good game by reliving yesterday's disaster and worrying about all the ways he will make a fool of himself today. In addition, Charlie is in constant turmoil with everyone, including Snoopy. How can he possibly concentrate and attend to what is going on around him during the game when he is attending to all those other thoughts in his head?

The usual approach of coaches and teachers is to try harder in the face of inconsistent performance and slow progress. Additional practice is spent on skills and getting back to the fundamentals.

However, athletes can never maximize their physical abilities until they learn to master their mental states. All athletes must develop their mental skills along with their physical skills if they are to reach their full potential. The athlete needs to be taught how to identify the factors that interfere with his/her performance to read bodily cues and to know which ones signal the loss of control, how to concentrate more fully for longer periods of time, how to "switch channels" and refocus when concentration lapses, what his/her optimal level of arousal is and how to reach it and maintain it throughout a competition, and how to set goals that can be evaluated in a systematic fashion. The coach is in the best position to incorporate these skills and strategies into the regular physical preparation for competition because he/she knows the athletes fairly well. He/she also knows the sport and the behavioral demands that are made on the athletes, how these may differ from position to position, and what behavioral responses specific situations within the sport may demand.

WHY TRAINING IN COGNITIVE SKILLS IS IMPORTANT

If you were told that the mind and body did not interact, you would most likely disagree. You could cite examples of how the cognitive perception of fear produces a racing heart, sweating, irregular breathing, muscular weakness, and so on. Or you might remember awakening from a nightmare and note that you are experiencing heart palpitations, sweating, respiratory distress, and other symptoms of panic. In point of fact, we literally *think with our muscles*! In fact, we cannot, under normal conditions, process cognitive thoughts without muscular action. Jacobson [1] demonstrated that over fifty years ago.

Our body is highly complex entity composed of a multitude of different yet highly integrated biological systems which promote effective interaction between our internal and external environments [2]. These highly differentiated systems are integrated and monitored by the nervous system. The nervous system is anatomically divided into the central and the peripheral nervous system. The brain and the spinal cord compose the central nervous system; the network of nerves connecting the various organs and systems of the body to the central nervous system makes up the peripheral nervous system. Thought and memory are the responsibility of the central nervous system. However, the entire nervous system allows integration of the mind and body to interpret consciously and unconsciously our external and internal environments. In sport and exercise a combination of reactions occur. Some of these responses are at the conscious level and some occur at a subconscious level As an example, if you perceive fear, your response may be to escape, either by running or to prepare to fight for your safety. This is Cannon's "fight or flight" response to fear or threat of one's well-being. Once this fear is perceived, other responses occur immediately, such as elevated blood pressure, increased blood flow to the muscles and vital organs, decreased blood flow to the digestive system, increased metabolism, etc. In short, all the bodily systems are geared for optimal function for protection and the cognitive focus is directed toward that end. These responses happen with real fear of your physical or mental well-being or with the cognitive (imagined) threat.

There are several critical factors that must be taken into consideration in understanding why the training of cognitive skills and strategies is effective in teaching athletes how to maximize their potential. According to Selye [3], stress is stress whether the stressor is perceived cognitively or is a real one such as exercise or heat. In either case, the body reacts in a predictable manner. Any stress, whether it be exercise, fear, worry, a deep emotional experience such as love, or whatever, preduces a similar physiological response. The body can only respond in a limited number of ways. During moments of panic or anxiety, we experience the same cardiorespiratory responses as when exercising: pounding of the heart, breathlessness, and subjective feelings of distress. Each individual must be able to recognize these responses and attribute them to the proper cause. In other words, when an athlete begins to notice these responses, he or she needs to identify the causal factors. If these responses are generated by the excitement and challenge of the anticipated competition and readiness to "get at them," there is generally no problem. However, if this same pattern of responses is attributed to worry and anxiety about how he or she will perform, then steps must be taken to keep things under control or decrements in performance will occur. Only the athlete can determine the stimulus that produces the response. They must be taught how to identfy the causes.

A second critical factor involves the fact that the mind/body is literal, that is it just knows that it has been there as in déjà vu. A distinction between whether you just thought about something, whether you dreamed about it, or whether you actually experienced it is difficult to make. The fact that the mind/body cannot make a clear distinction between just thinking about doing something and actually doing it will have particular implications for some of the things I will discuss later.

The third critical factor relates to the optimal level of arousal needed for maximal performance. Each individual has to determine his or her optimal level of arousal, know how to reach it, and how to maintain it in order to produce consistent performance. Insufficient arousal produces less than maximal performance and usually results in the classic upsets we observe in sport on occasion. If an individual athlete or a team goes into a competition with the odds hgihly in their favor, they might not be sufficiently aroused to produce their best performance, resulting in a loss. On the other hand, too much arousal produces a poor performance as well with some sports and some positions in a particular sport being affected to a greater extent then others. The real challenge is to help each athlete find his or her optimal level and to teach each individual how to maintain that over time.

An additional critical factor regarding why cognitive training assists athletes in maximizing their performance is the fact that stress or arousal can be either chronic or acute, general or situational. Identification of situationally specific arousal in sport is fairly easy. When the athlete can associate specific responses to competitive sport situations, it is much easier to learn to control them.

Another factor that has relevance for cognitive training concerns the application of the skills and strategies that are learned. If an athlete can only use them under ideal situations and not when he or she needs them, they are not worth the time spent to learn them. They must be learned and practiced to the same degree of proficiency as any physical skill so that they can be utilized when needed.

Finally, Bandura's [4] self-efficacy model for psychotherapeutic change provides further support for cognitive training. According to Bandura, "cognitive processes mediate change but . . . cognitive events are induced and altered most readily by experiencing mastery arising from effective performance." Sport performance provides instant feedback with regard to experiencing masterly arising from effective performance. The association of cognitive skills with effective performance can be made immediately when it occurs. This serves to reinforce the cognitive control in hopes of consistent and continued improvement of performance. The athlete can see the relevancy of what is being learned.

LEARNING PROGRESSIONS FOR COGNITIVE SKILLS AND STRATEGIES

Once the athlete has learned the relationship between worry, anxiety, and performance and has observed the difference between performance without worry and anxiety compared to that accompanied by worry and anxiety, he or she is ready to take steps to control those factors that interfere. The first step is to identify the pattern of somatic and cognitive responses that occur when worry and anxiety begin. Some of the immediate somatic cues are palpitations of the heart, muscle tension, sense of weakness and fatigue, irritability, cotton mouth, cold clammy hands and feet, butterflies in the stomach, desire to urinate, visual distortions, trembling and twitches in muscles, flushed face, voice distortion, nausea and vomiting, diarrhea, hyperventilation, and increased heart rate, blood pressure, and respiration. Some of the cognitive signals are sense of confusion, forgetting details, inability to concentrate, resorting to old habits, and inability to make decisions. Obviously, if any one individual had all of these symptoms, he or she would not be able to function at all. Each athlete has to learn his or her particular pattern of responses to overarousal resulting from worry and anxiety about the upcoming performance. Athletes will differ with regard to how much their performance is affected; therefore, it is essential that they learn to identify the response associated with anxiety and begin to regulate their arousal before it gets out of control.

As indicated earlier, the mind/body has only a limited number of ways of responding to stimulation. As a result, the response pattern is generally the same. Athletes must learn to evaluate their self-thoughts and perceptions in order to determine whether the response pattern is resulting from the excitement and anticipation of the challenge and is their usual state of optimal arousal or whether it is produced by worry and fear about how they will perform. In order to determine this, athletes need to get to know themselves and to be able to read their bodily signals. Further, they need to keep a diary on a regular basis so they can, in retrospect, analyze how they performed in relation to how they felt prior to performance. In this way, they can begin to determine the pattern of response that leads to an exceptional performance as well as the pattern of responses and feelings that produce an inferior performance. Good performances and bad performances are not just lucky and unlucky situations; they are caused. Once the pattern has been established, each athlete can begin to set the stage for a good performance. There is no assurance that the performance will always be a good one; however, the probability of a good one occurring is much greater. From that point the athlete needs to learn skills and strategies that will assist in regulating responses that lead to poor performance.

Relaxation

When a muscle is tense, it is contracted or shortened. This contraction involves nerves as well with about half of the nerves in the body being used to alert the muscles to respond while the other half carry messages to the brain. The activity of the nerves, which is electrical in nature, moves along the muscle like a wave with a rapid discharge rate. When this rate increases greatly, there is a high nerve tension and the muscles can become rigid. Our problem, however, is that human nerve circuits have no automatic regulators. There are no signals to alert you to too much tension.

Muscle tissue works in one direction; it can only pull which it does by shortening and thickening itself. Consequently, the voluntary muscles in animals are arranged in pairs. When a muscle tightens, its opposite of the pair sets up a counter tension to hold the segment of the body in place. This double pull can build up formidable heights of tension over much of the body yet remain unidentified by most people. The double pull explains why you can be scared stiff, why you can become rigid with anger, unable to move with stage fright, unable to speak, etc. It also explains why you may shoot air balls, blow a short putt, pass with too much force, overhit a tennis ball, mistime a strategic move, and so on. The principle of the double pull has great significance for athletes. When you watch athletes who move effortlessly, they are using the proper form. The proper form involves using just the right amount of tension necessary to do the skill, to move the body in the most efficient manner with the least amount of energy. Too much muscular tension interferes with the execution of skill. Excessive muscular tension can be triggered by mental input that is generated by worry and anxiety. Obviously, when the nerve pathways are occupied by impulses alerting the system to "fight or flight," the impulses necessary for skillful, coordinated movement are inhibited to some degree. The more muscular tension in the muscle, the more difficult it is to execute good form in any type of movement.

Total relaxation means letting go and doing absolutely nothing with your muscles. Although muscles cannot be switched off completely, they can be brought down nicely to an idling speed. You may be wondering why an athlete would want to be completely relaxed. What has relaxation got to do with competitive sport? Athletes need muscular tension and arousal to perform; some need maximal tension to accomplish their sport. In training the muscles to relax, the athlete develops a much greater sensitivity to his/her bodily feelings and responses. Once you learn to attend to somatic responses and to associate these with certain types of behavior and performance, you learn to regulate tension to deal with the environment actively and effectively.

Once you have learned the skill, relaxation techniques can be used to lower general muscular tension under any conditions where you are producing too much. Relaxation will assist in removing localized tension such as that occurring with headaches and lower back pain. It can facilitate recovery when you have only a short time to rest. Relaxation also promotes sleep onset and reduces insomnia problems that plague many athletes prior to competition. Probably the most important contribution that relaxation can make to an athlete is to teach regulation of muscular tension so that nerve path ways to the muscle are never overcharged.

In general, the techniques of relaxation can be divided into two categories. In the first category the techniques that focus on the somatic aspects of those that are considered, "muscle to mind." Jacobson's [5] scientific neuromuscular relaxation or progressive relaxation would fall under this category. The objective is to train the muscles to become sensitive to any level of tension. You learn this by generating as much tension as possible, letting go, and studying the difference as you progress through muscle groups. The second caretory of techniques include the cognitive or mental approaches to relaxation; these work from the "mind to the muscle." Benson's relaxation response, meditation, autogenic training, and imagery all approach relaxation from the cognitive perspective. Either approach is effective; the point is to disrupt the stimulus-response pattern at some point in the cycle. Whether you focus your attention on the efferent portion of the central nervous system from brain to muscle or whether you focus on afferent portion, reducing the stimulation to the brain, is immaterial. Reducing the sensation in either half of the circuit will interrupt the circuit of stimulation necessary to produce muscular tension.

Self-Thoughts and Self-Talk

Each of us is continuously engaging in self-talk or our own internal cognitive processing. Most of us go beyond what is occurring right here and now in our thought processing. Our cognitions go beyond what the situation is providing in that they trigger memories of what has happened in the past in similar situations and other associations that have nothing to do specifically with what is currently going on. We tend to ruminate about how that similar situation affected us, what we did about it, and what the previous outcome was. Beyond that we jump ahead and begin to imagine how the present situation will go and begin to dwell on the anticipated outcome before it occurs. Obviously, such thought associations can sometimes run away and lead to disasterous consequences. When these thought patterns are generated, they prevent focusing the attention on what is happening and about to happen within the competitive experience. Concentration is impossible when the "programmer' is already overloaded with irrelevant thoughts that disrupt rather than enhance performance.

Athletes must be taught to become aware of their self-thoughts and self-talk. Once they develop this awareness, they can begin to identify those that increase and encourage worry and anxiety. Once these are identified, athletes can develop strategies for changing negative thoughts to positive ones. They can learn to let negative thoughts pass on through when they do occur and refocus to positive self-coaching ones. When this is learned, situations will never develop into panic ones accompanied by a sense of being out of control.

Goal setting, which we will discuss later, is closely related to self-talk and can provide a positive source of self-statements when the goals are specific to the practice or performance. Positive self-talk regarding specific goals also focuses concentration on the here and now.

Our beliefs and expectancies about the outcome of the performance have a great deal to do with the actual outcome of the event. Self-fulfilling prophecies are numerous in sports performance. As beliefs about the limits of our performance change, the limits of our performance actually change as well. A classic example of a psychological barrier in sport performance is breaking the sub-four-minute mile. Once Roger Bannister demonstrated that it was possible, over 50 runners managed to accomplish the feat in the next couple years. Psychological knowledge of what is possible has a great deal to do with what one can accomplish.

Concentration and Attentional Focus

One of the major causes of inconsistency in performance is lack of concentration. Lapses in concentration cause all sorts of mental errors and mistakes. Actually, concentration is just paying attention to what you are doing or about to do; however, it is a skill that has to be learned and must be practiced regularly to maintain. Concentration involves being able to attend to what is going on over time without a lapse in your attention. If you are not focused 100 percent on what you are doing, your performance cannot be maximal. When you are concentrating and giving your undivided attention to the task at hand, you are aware of nothing else.

An athlete's attention may be spread over many relevant cues, or it can be concentrated on a specific one. The nature of the sport or the specific demands of a particular position will alter the dimensions of concentration. In most sports no single cue demands the focus of attention for extended periods of time. While the athlete's attention is selective, what is being selected may change rapidly from one moment to the next. As the attentional focus increases on what is going on around the athlete in sport, the attention directed to the self will diminish. However, if the focus of attention stays on the self—that is, on how worried and anxious you are about performing—then the attention directed to what is going on around you will diminish. This is perhaps the main cause of lack of concentration observed in sport. Athletes need to learn how to shift attention from the self to the sports environment as the situation may demand.

In sport, the external or environmental focus includes the immediate processing of information that is being picked up by the eyes and ears. The self-focus includes such things as the physiological responses to exertion and/or to worry and anxiety. Many athletes may be self-focused prior to the competition but shift to external focus as the action begins. Others do not have the ability to shift as easily and take some time to adjust to the pace of the game. A classic example of inability to shift attention is when an athlete makes a mistake and continues to be preoccupied with that. If the concentration is not focused on what is happening or about to happen additional mistakes will be made.

Maximal sport performance occurs when intense concentration of attention is focused on a limited stimulus field where only relevant cues are processed from the multitude available. All irrelevant stimuli are ignored. Peak performance occurs when you voluntarily concentrate (just let it happen) on the relevant cues in the game and perceive them to demand a response that is within your ability. That is, the challenge of the situation must match your perception of ability in order to maintain concentration over time. If the challenge is greater than the perceived ability, concentration will lapse as you begin to worry about that. On the other hand, if your skills are beyond the challenge, you may not be able to maintain sufficient arousal to stay concentrated. This results in the classic upsets we see in sport season after season. The relationship between the balance of challenge and skills and sustained concentration has been observed not only in sport but in many other pursuits as well.

Certain positions in specific sports or specific tasks in some sports require one type of attentional focus while other positions and sports demand a different type. A narrow focus of attention, looking at one thing or focusing on a relatively small area, is required in target sports, shooting sports, foul shooting, kicking a field goal, or kicking for an extra point. On the other hand, a broad focus of attention is required in most team games where you have to be aware of your opponents, your teammates, and the ball.

Further, most team sports require the ability to shift back and forth from a broad to narrow focus of attention, whereas most closed skills demand a narrow focus throughout the contest. Team sport athletes need to learn to adjust and change their focus of attention much as a zoom lens in a camera.

Mental errors are generally caused by lack of concentration which can result from anxiety, worry, or laziness. Many times coaches cause mental errors when they attempt to coach from the sidelines. If an athlete is trying to concentrate on what is going on within the game, he or she cannot attend to what the coach is saying at the same time. Coaches need to realize that coaching from the sidelines is generally counterproductive because it disrupts concentration.

Imagery, Visualization, or Mental Practice

Using your imagination or visualizing in your mind's eye is a powerful tool that you can use to improve anything and everything. Using imagery in sport is of particular importance because you literally "think with your muscles." For full benefit, it is important to learn how to control and concentrate on imagery training. Most of us daydream and reexperience situations in a haphazard manner, letting thoughts pass in and out and wander.

Brown [6], in her book, *Supermind*, discussed the use of imagination as the ultimate energy in accomplishing things. She said that imagination was the most neglected and underdeveloped ability of humans. Imagination can recreate the past in great detail or transform it to fit the emotional states desired. It can project into the future, solve problems, gain relief from mental pressures, assist in learning and maximizing performance, and entertain us.

Most athletes have discovered the use of imagery as a means to improving their performance; however, few have been given instructions and guidance in ways to gain all the potential that it might offer. Imagery involves recalling from memory pieces of information stored there from all types of experiences and reshaping them into a meaningful reverie via a thought process. Inasmuch as experiences can be remembered through several sense organs, you may be able to see, taste, hear, feel, or experience other sensory stimuli kinesthetically. Many athletes do not "see" as such in their mind's eye. Their images are not visual but more kinesthetical in that they "feel" themselves executing their skills. Becoming more aware of all dimensions of the performance experience is essential in providing the necessary cues for practicing imagery. The déjà vu effect, the feeling of having been there before, is apparent in using imagery. When an action is imagined the central nervous system sends impulses in a pattern associated with that action. The stimulation that is generated by imagining is manifested bodily in the neurological patterns generating low levels of muscular response. The more the skill is imagined, the more efficient and effective subsequent imagery or action becomes. Using this strategy, you can practice what you have already learned to improve your performance or you can increase your speed of learning by adding mental practice.

Brown [6], indicated that there were two remarkable benefits of imagery that have been scientifically validated but not systematically used to increase human performance. First, the more specific and detailed the image, the more specific the effect. That is, cognitively, you can excite and generate impulses that are specific to the pattern of response necessary to produce the movement. Secondly imagining makes the body work; mental images direct and activate the neurological patterning of nerves to make the body respond exactly the way the image directs it. This effect has tremendous implications for athletes. If you concentrate and imagine that you are executing your sport skill just as you would like, you are not only imagining, you are preparing your body to perform. Your nerves, muscles, heart, breathing, and sympathetic nervous system all integrate with the initial cognitive image to see/feel yourself accomplishing your performance.

Another positive benefit of imagery is that of being able to imagine situations and practice all types of options in sports performance that you cannot possibly accomplish in practice. As an example, if you have no practice partner who can challenge you, you can imagine that you are competing against someone much better than you to improve your game. Or, as a goalie, you may not be able to have your teammates shoot every type of shot at goal, but you can imagine all of those in your head and practice stopping them. In fact, you can practice anything in your mind's eye and can prepare in a way that is not always possible in physical practice. You can set up all types of conditions and situations in your head with mental imagery that you cannot possibly structure in a real life practice. You can prepare for anything.

Mental imagery is generally more effective with the highly skilled athlete; however, it can be used at any skill level. The more cues and experience you have in the physical practice, the more effective the imagery will be. Imagery is easier to practice in those sports where the execution of the skills takes place in similar and controlled situations. Individual sports are more conducive to imagery practice because they do not involve actions of teammates or opponents in some cases. Individual sports such as gymnastics, diving, skating, and the like are ideal sports for mental imagery. Team sports involve many additional dimensions but can be practiced in your mind's eye as well. Imagery can be used to practice specific plays, offenses, or defenses. Mental practice, in combination with physical practice, provides the best method of preparation for competition. Mental practice is not a substitute for physical practice; however, it can enhance both the amount and the quality of physical practice.

In mental imagery, the sequence of movements should be rehearsed just as desired in performance, at the same pace and from beginning to end. All dimensions of the performance and all the possible sensory cues should be incorporated. The mental rehearsal should be equal to or better than previous performances, not perfect. If perfect performance is rehearsed, failure to perform up to the expectancy is bound to occur as perfection occurs so infrequently in sport. However, when mentally rehearsing target sports such as shooting, archery, basketball shooting, field goals, etc., successful accomplishment of the task should be visualized.

Reexperiencing a successful performance as soon as possible after it occurred is a good way to learn to associate the mind/body integration that is required to execute at a high level. Some athletes find that "walking through" or mimicing many of the movements as they imagine executing them also increases the benefits of imagery. Word cues and self-thoughts will assist in focusing your imagery during mental rehearsal as well. Imagery can be used effectively when injured or unable to physically perform; athletes report they maintain their skill level at a fairly high level in this manner.

As one becomes more proficient in the skill of imagery, unlimited ways of practicing and preparing for every detail and every aspect of sport performance will be discovered. Competitions can be prepared for by actually playing them ahead of time in the mind's eye. The first time you experience déjà vu that results from having "been there before" in your mind's eye, you will realize the great benefits of mental imagery rehearsal for anything and everything that you hope to accomplish. Practicing this skill allows you to remember things of the past, to work on things that are in the present, and to project into the future in preparation for events that are yet to happen. It is one of the effective ways of learning and improving and preparing for the application of them in a dynamic setting.

Motivation through Goal Setting

Goal setting is simply identifying what you are trying to do or to accomplish and is viewed primarily as a mechanism for motivation. Research in goal setting during the decade of the 1970s has generated several conclusions. The positive effect of goal setting on performance is one of the most replicable findings in the psychological literature [7]. The beneficial effects that goal setting has on performance are explained by four mechanisms of motivation: directing action, mobilizing effort, persisting with effort over time, and generating motivation to develop relevant and alternative strategies for attaining goals. Those who set difficult and challenging goals outperform those who set "do your best" goals or easy ones. Goals appear to motivate performance more successfully when they are stated in specific quantitative terms or actions rather than "trying harder."

Goals can be viewed as regulators of motivation; the importance of establishing goals cannot be understated. All dimensions of motivation, attentional focus, effort put forth, the persistence of effort, and continued development of relevant strategies to attain goals are structured through goal setting. What one is trying to accomplish should be clearly delineated for training, for practice, and for competition by stating goals specific to each of those conditions.

Athletes should set their own goals in collaboration with their coaches and teammates. Goals should be process oriented, not just stated in terms of outcomes. That is, goals should be specific to what one has to do to win rather than just setting the goal to win. Major goals may have several other related goals. If the goal of improving running by reducing time over distance was stated, other goals to assist in attainment might involve weight loss or weight training. Goals should be stated in positive terms that can be evaluated so that one will know when they are attained. They must be stated in relation to what the current level of accomplishment is so that they are realistic. In other words, all goals should be related to performances that are attainable.

Goals should be established for different time schedules as well as for different components leading to attainment. Immediate goals can be structured for an upcoming practice, for the week, or for preseason. Other goals can focus on the season or for some intermediate aspect of the long-range plan. The long-term goals will involve those things desired over a competitive career. With such a plan, goal setting can structure a course of action for individuals, for the team, and for the coach. Goal setting can provide guidelines for training, and for competition. Establishing realistic, meaningful, measureable goals for all involved can eliminate motivation problems, and everyone will know specifically what they are trying to accomplish. As immediate and intermediate goals are attained, the positive feedback will reinforce the motivation to persist toward the attainment of long-term goals. Keep in mind that success comes in many ways other than winning. If you plan for experiencing success along the way, winning will generally take care of itself.

MONITORING PROGRESS IN LEARNING COGNITIVE SKILLS AND STRATEGIES

Keeping a daily log of your progress in practicing and applying cognitive skills and strategies is the best way to monitor your progress [8]. Eventually you should be able to observe a pattern of behavior and preparation that leads to a good performance or a pattern that leads to a poor performance. In this way an understanding of what contributes to good performance can be gained. You can learn how to prepare consistently for competition by including all the preparations that have led to previous good performances, thus setting the stage for what will hopefully be another good one.

Goal setting at all levels should be included in your log, starting with the long term, followed by the intermediate and short-term goals that will lead to attainment of the long-term goal.

Everything that you feel influences your performance in any way should be recorded on a daily basis. Your daily training and practice goals should be stated and evaluated with regard to whether you met them or not. Keeping a dietary record is also a good idea, particularly if you are trying to reach or maintain a certain weight. You may discover that certain foods have less than a positive effect on your performance when you keep a daily record.

Develop the habit of writing down thoughts and feelings about everything involving participation. These might include reactions to teammates, coaches, practices, playing time, etc. In this way you may discover a response pattern that tends to interfere with your performance and can begin to do something about it.

A systematic record of how and what types of relaxation techniques you practice and when you practice and use them will also be helpful. Make notes concerning how your sleeping pattern is influenced by relaxation. You can also monitor your progress in improving concentration by keeping a record of how well you are able to direct your attentional focus, maintain it, and regain it when it lapses. Your use of imagery, visualization, and mental rehearsal should also be recorded on a regular basis in order to evaluate the effectiveness.

Each day you should evaluate your performance at practice or at competition so that you can compare what you have done in preparation with how well you perform. In this manner you can determine the relationship of what you do and how you perform. You will see that you can develop control of your behavior as it relates to all aspects of your performance.

It may take weeks, months, and even years of systematic effort to integrate and fine tune all the necessary components to maximize performance potential. The more you learn about how to control and regulate your responses to adjust for optimal arousal, the greater your success. Incorporating cognitive skills and strategies with your physical practice will not ensure an Olympic gold medal; however, you can be sure that you will maintain a more consistent performance record and come closer to performing at your potential under any and all conditions.

REFERENCES

1. Jacobson, E. Electrical measures of neuromuscular states during mental activities. *Am. J. Physio.*, *91*, 567, 1930.
2. Benson, H. *The Mind/Body Effect*. New York: Simon and Shuster, 1979.
3. Selye, H. *The Stress of Life*. New York: McGraw-Hill, 1956.
4. Bandura, A. Self-efficiency: Toward a unifying theory of behavioral change. *Psychol. Rev.*, *84*, 191, 1977.
5. Jacobson, E. *You Must Relax*. New York: McGraw-Hill, 1976.
6. Brown, B. *Supermind*. New York: Harper & Row, 1980.
7. Locke, E. A., Shaw, K. N., Saari, L. M. and Latham, G. P. Goal setting and task performance: 1969-1980. *Psychol. Bul.*, *90*, 125, 1981.
8. Harris, D., and Harris, B. *The Athlete's Guide to Sports Psychology: Mental Skills for Physical People*. West Point: Leisure Press, 1983.

CHAPTER 11

A Preliminary Study of Elite Adolescent Women Athletes and Their Attitudes toward Training and Femininity

Jerry R. May, Tracy L. Veach, Denise Daily-McKee, and George Furman

The psychological makeup of women and the impact of sports on them is an often-discussed topic by the media, coaches, parents, and women themselves. Athletics and masculinity traditionally have been linked in the public's mind. In order to participate and excell in sports, one must possess the masculine characteristics of being tough, competitive, and hard-driving, or so goes the myth. Berlin [1] pointed out that the female who participates in athletics often has her womanhood or femininity questioned. This is indeed unfortunate.

There is some evidence that attitudes of the general public and women athletes themselves are improving regarding women's involvement in sports. Snyder and Spreiter [2] have found that high-school women athletes actually rate themselves as equal or even more feminine than their nonathletic counterparts. Harris [3] reported that physically inactive college women have poorer self-images than physically active women. In fact, female college athletes are significantly more assertive, more conscientious, and more venturesome

The Elite Athlete, edited by N. K. Butts, T. T. Gushiken, and B. Zarins. Copyright © 1985 by Spectrum Publications, Inc.

and independent than their nonathletic counterparts [4]. Thus, there is some change taking place with respect to how women feel about being athletes and possibly an attitudinal shift among society in its beliefs about the role of women in sports. One factor in this change may be due to a change in our athlete role models. The role models for most social and cultural attitudes are usually developed from the acceptance of celebrities who have excelled in their particular field. Until shifts in attitude occur in elite women athletes, little consistent and broad-ranging change can be expected in public opinion. The present pilot study addresses the issue of some of the psychological attitudes of elite female athletes who are women's role models. These women's attitudes will be an important factor in cultural attitude change.

SUBJECT POPULATION

One hundred and sixteen elite female athletes who attended training camps at the U.S. Olympic Center in Squaw Valley, California, participated in the study. The women were members of national teams in synchronized swimming, modern rhythmic gymnastics, track, cross-country running, alpine skiing, basketball, and

Table 11.1. Background on Female Athlete Respondents

Type of Sport	N	Age**		Years in Competition**	
		Mean	SD	Mean	SD
Synchronized Swimming	63	15.37	1.76	4.98	1.69
Modern Rhythmic Gymnastics	18	19.50	5.65	4.33	4.73
Track, Cross-country Running	22	19.14	3.14	4.77	2.35
Other*	13	18.92	2.22	8.08	3.26
All	116	17.12	3.52	5.17	2.94

*Members of U.S. Alpine Ski Team, National Basketball Team, and U.S. Figure Skating Team.
**Using Analysis of Variance (ANOVA), both age and year of competition differ by sport. (F = 15.96, $P < .001$; F = 5.16, $P < .002$, respectively)

figure skating. Table 11.1 provides the demographic background on the female athletes. The category entitled, "Other" includes the women in skiing, basketball, and figure skating.

METHODS

Data were collected from questionnaires distributed after a lecture to the athlete groups. Questions were designed to elicit the individual's attitudes regarding dating behavior, femininity, perceptions of peers, perceptions of training effects on femininity, attitudes toward masculine-looking muscles, and the effects of menstruation on athletic performance.

RESULTS

Comparisons of the athlete groups revealed no statistically significant differences for the attitude variables under study. Both age and years in competition, however, did differ by sport (see Table 11.1). Synchronized swimmers were younger, and the aggregate group of skiers, skaters, and basketball players had more competitive experience.

Data on how training effects dating behavior for elite female athletes is presented in Table 11.2. A large number of respondents felt training reduced dating. A larger group, however, reported no perceived change in dating behavior as a result of being an athlete. A small percentage believed that it enhanced their dating behavior. Those athletes reporting reduced dating behavior reported the reason was not a femininity issue but a lack of time.

Table 11.2. Training Effects on Dating Behavior of Female Athletes

Training Results	Frequency	Percentage
No response	6	5.2
More dates	14	12.1
Fewer dates	44	37.9
No change	52	44.8
	116	100.0

Table 11.3. Female Athletes' Perception of
How Peers (Social Contacts) View Femininity
of Women Athletes

Athletes' Perception	Frequency	Percentage
No response	5	4.3
More feminine	12	10.3
Less feminine	14	12.1
No difference	85	73.3
	116	100.0

Table 11.3 presents the data of how female athletes perceive their peers (social contacts) view the femininity of women athletes compared to their nonathletic counterparts. The majority of respondents believed being an athlete does not influence the perception of others with regard to their femininity. A small percentage believed that they are perceived as either more feminine or less feminine.

The data on the individual female athlete's perception of training effects on femininity or masculinity are presented in Table 11.4. Specifically, the majority felt training does not lead to development of masculine-looking muscles. Approximately one-fourth of the athletes believed training did result in masculine-looking muscles, mostly from the synchronized swimming group and the modern rhythmic gymnastics team. It is interesting that although individuals did perceive some increased in muscle development, the majority viewed it as positive or were indifferent (see Table 11.5). In fact, only a small percentage viewed it as a negative training consequence.

Table 11.4. Female Athletes' Perception of Training
Effects on Femininity/Masculinity

Training Results in Masculine Appearance (muscle development)	Frequency	Percentage
Yes	25	21.5
No	85	73.3
Sometimes	1	.9
No response	5	4.3
	116	100.0

Table 11.5. Female Athletes' Attitude toward
"Masculine-Looking Muscles" as an Aspect of
Their Olympic Training

Attitude toward Muscles	Frequency	Percentage
No response	7	6
Positive	63	54.3
Negative	8	6.9
Indifferent	38	32.8
	116	100.0

A unique characteristic of women athletes is the influence of menstruation on athletic performance. Menstruation was found to have a major effect on mood. Sixty percent of the women reported mood changes during the menstrual cycle. Interestingly, the effects of these mood changes on athletic performance was quite minimal (see Table 11.6). Most women reported that the mood changes resulting from menstruation had no effect. Approximately one-fourth of the women did report some negative effect on their performance. Unexpectedly, a small percentage of the women reported a positive change.

DISCUSSION

In general, the young elite women athletes in the study have a positive self-concept about their participation in sports. They believe themselves to be at least as feminine as their nonathletic counterparts and possess a positive body image.

Table 11.6. Emotional Effects of Menstruation
and Its Influence upon Athletic Performance

Effect on Performance	Frequency	Percentage
No response	16	13.8
Positive	6	5.2
No change	66	56.9
Negative	28	24.1
	116	100.0

The question of loss of femininity may no longer be an important variable for women athletes. Most important is the fact that young women felt good about themselves, and their athletic interests and activities need not be tied to either masculinity or femininity. Well-adjusted individuals commonly report feeling comfortable with the cuturally determined "masculine" or "feminine" characteristics as part of their personality. It is unfortunate that our society makes such a distinction. It may well be that eventually sporting activities will play a role in breaking down some of this dichotomy. In clinical work, one of the authors (J. May) has found these female athletes to be highly motivated and confident of themselves as individuals.

Training and competitive schedules do interfere with dating behavior for some athletes, but this is due to the priority given to their sport and the time commitment required by training. Remember that these young women are elite athletes who spend four to eight hours per day practicing their chosen sport in addition to attending school. The authors have observed this same reduction in dating behavior with male athletes and, therefore, do not view it as being a sex-linked characteristic.

It is believed that female athletes are becoming more accepted today and are feeling more accepted. Athletic competition can be a positive experience in a woman's developmental process. Attitudes regarding women in sports stem from existing female athlete role models and cultural expectations. As the self-concept of elite role model women improves, so will the general public's perception of women in sports. The problems encountered and the coping strategies for female athletes appear similar to those of males and, therefore, do not need to be explained by sex. Hopefully, there will be a continued increase in the acceptance of women in sports by men and women of the general population.

The psychologists, physicians, and coaches can play an active role in disseminating the information regarding the positive changes toward being a woman athlete. Encouragement can be given to schools, parents, and young girls that involvement in physical activities and competitive sports can lead to improved self-image, confidence, enjoyment, and excitement in a young girl's life. Femininity can be maintained, and if it is not, it is probably not a function of one's participation in sports activities but other significant life influences. Maybe the most important fact is that if a young girl chooses to develop certain "masculine" characteristics, it does not bother her as much as it used to in the past and these young women need not be stereotyped.

ACKNOWLEDGMENTS

Funding for the project was provided in part by the U.S. Olympic Sports Medicine Program and Grant #14514, Psychiatry Education Branch, National Institutes of Mental Health.

REFERENCES

1. Berlin, P. The woman athlete. In E. W. Gerber, J. Felshin, P. Berlin, W. Wyrish (Eds.), *The American Woman in Sport*. Reading, MA.: Eddison-Wesley, 1974.
2. Snyder, E. D., and Spreiter, E. *Social aspects of sports*. Englewood Cliffs, NJ, Prentice Hall, Inc., 1978.
3. Harris, D. Personal communication, University of Pennsylvania, 1980.
4. King, J. P., and Chi, P. S. Social structure, sex roles, and personality: Comparison of male-female athletes-non-athletes. In J. H. Goldstein (Ed.), *Sports, Games, and Play*. Hillsdale, NJ: Lawrence Erlbaum Assoc., 1979.

CHAPTER **12**

The Effects of Life Change on Injuries, Illness, and Performance in Elite Athletes

Jerry R. May, Tracy L. Veach, Scott W. Southard,
and Michael W. Herring

LITERATURE REVIEW

Psychological factors in injury, illness, and performance in athletic events are becoming a more frequently discussed topic. Rosenblum [1] reported that it is important that all of those involved in the training and care of athletes be aware of emotional conditions that lead to injuries, both physical and psychological, as well as conditions which interfere with performance and effectiveness. Green, Gabrielsen, Hall, and O'Heir [2] observed that the majority of swimming pool accidents in their study resulted from a lack of good judgment and common sense rather than from intoxication or pool structural deficiencies. Many individuals agree that this is an important aspect of sports medicine, but very little systematic research has been conducted.

Pioneering work by Holmes and Rahe [3] has demonstrated that life events may have direct psychological and physical consequences

Reprinted from *Ski Coach* 4(6), 1983, by permission.

for the individual in the general population. The conclusions of Holmes and Rahe are well accepted, and knowledge of life events and their impact on illness and injury has been increased. Bramwell, Masuda, Wagner, and Holmes [4] expanded this early research into the area of life stresses and athletic injuries. They modified the life-change scale to athletic populations and investigated the relationship between athletic injuries and life change among football players on the University of Washington varsity football team. Findings indicated that the injured group of athletes had a signigicant higher life stress level than the noninjured group. Coddington and Troxell [5] conducted a similar study on high-school football players employing a life events scale for adolescents. They reported significant differences between the injured and noninjured athletes for the factors of family events and object loss. Six players reported divorce of their parents, and four players reported death of a parent. They concluded that the risk of injuries for these players was five times greater than for those reporting no such loss.

More recently, Seese [6], employing the Life Experiences Survey developed by Sarason, Johnson, and Siegel [7], studied the effects of life experiences on football injuries. In particular, Seese was interested in examining the relationship of desirable and undesirable events to athletic injuries. A positive correlation was found between life change and subsequent athletic injuries. However, the importance of positive versus negative life-change events did not reveal any differences in relationship to the onset of injuries.

Unfortunately to date the only sport investigated has been football. The present study was developed to investigate the effect of life events change on illness, injury, and performance in elite athletes. Various athlete groups, rather than one unified group, were examined. A major hypothesis was that life events predict the onset of illness and injury. Type of illness and injury, as well as frequency, duration, and severity, were also investigated. Another hypothesis was that change in life events would negatively influence athletic performance outcomes. A third hypothesis predicted that positive and negative life events would be differentially related to onset of illness and injury. Finally, it was of interest to determine if specific athletic groups experienced different levels of change.

MATERIALS AND METHODS

Ninety-seven elite male and female athletes representing primarily five sports (biathalon, race walking, figure skating, gymnastics, and basketball) attending the Sports Medicine Program at the Olympic

Training Center in Squaw Valley, California, participated in the study.

The amount of life change experienced by the athletes was assessed by use of the Social Athletic Readjustment Rating Questionnaire (SARRQ) with slight scoring modifications developed by Bramwell et al. [4]. The athletes were surveyed on the presence or frequency of life-change events in each of two six-month periods preceding this administration. Life-change events included items such as divorce, death of spouse, conflict with coach, and other potentially stressful changes in living and training circumstances.

One year later, each athlete was mailed a Health, Injury, Illness and Performance Survey (HIPS), developed by modifying the health history questionnaire used by Christensen [8]. Injuries and illnesses were grouped under 26 categories of organ systems, with specific diseases of that organ system listed as clarifying examples. *Frequency* of each health problem was obtained from the athlete's reports of the number of separate occurrences of each health problem, for the year prior to HIPS administration.

Duration of a problem was measured by total number of days each problem lasted, and *severity* was assessed by the athlete's own rating of a problem as minor, moderate, or severe, for the entire year prior to HIPS administration.

Self-reported performance data (national and regional rankings) on these elite athletes were also collected on the HIPS questionnaire to assess the impact of life-change events on performance.

The HIPS questionnaire mailing produced a 61% return response. The timing of the HIPS follow-up one year after the original SARRQ data collection means that the data on injury, illness, and performance relates approximately to the year immediately following administration of the SARRQ. Data from these surveys were then coded and analyzed using statistical routines from the Statistical Package from the Social Sciences (SPSS).

RESULTS

Table 12.1 provides a breakdown of the life-change data that was obtained. Analysis of variance (ANOVA) shows that athletes' mean scores do differ significantly by type of sport ($F = 2.48$; $p < .05$). Basketball players are clearly the group with the highest amount of reported life change. This is not too surprising given their younger ages and the fact that most have recently entered college. Analyses of the demographics found that age was, in fact, significantly related

Table 12.1   Life-Change Scores by Type of Sport

Sport		Life-Change Score	
	n	Mean	Standard Deviation
Gymnastics	15	523	220
Figure Skating	9	371	157
Basketball	12	773	236
Biathalon	28	452	285
Race Walking	28	523	470

to type of sport. Frequently reported life-change events include changes in school, team participation, and similar stresses. The race-walking and biathalon athletes are older and report life changes more related to occupational and financial events (e.g., house, mortgage, etc.). Indeed, most of the differences between the groups are probably a function of age differences rather than sport per se.

A major hypothesis is that life-change scores will be predictive of subsequent health, injury, and performance problems in athletes. Table 12.2 shows the specific health problems that are significantly correlated with the life-change scores. These data clearly support the hypothesis predicting subsequent problems for athletes with higher reported life-change scores. Considering the particular group of athletes studied, it is not too surprising to find musculoskeletal problems of the legs and feet to be a somatic focus of potential stressful life events. The reported use of nonprescription substances, however, was not as expected. All three measures of nonprescription drug use (frequency, duration, and severity) were significantly related to life-change events. Unfortunately, the present survey did not require respondents to list the specific substances. Consequently, it is not clear what specific self-medicative patterns may be associated with life-change stresses.

The grouping of health problems is also very interesting. These are largely problems that could be expected to be sensitive or reactive to high-stress levels (i.e., psychosomatic type problems). Frequency of health problem appears to be most sensitive to life-change events, although duration and severity are also related to some type of problems.

Not surprisingly, many of the health problems are related to type of sport. Table 12.3 shows those problems where ANOVA techniques significantly differentiated athlete groups as to mean frequency and duration of the health problem. Obviously, the

Table 12.2 Correlations between Life-Change Scores and the Frequency, Duration, and Severity of Health Problems (N = 59)

Problems	Correlation Coefficients		
	Frequency	Duration	Severity[1]
Headaches	.31**	.01	.26
Respiratory	.07	.31*	.22
Digestive		.06	.27
Musculoskeletal-arms		−.03	.08
Musculoskeletal-legs and feet	.33**	.48**	.37*
Skin	−.26* #	−.12	.20
Anxiety	.26*	.10	.22
Weight gain/loss	.23*	.14	.25
Substance use (non-prescription)	.46**	.32*	.43*

*$p<.05$
**$p<.01$
#Contrary to hypothesis, but statistically significant.
[1] Severity correlations were calculated from eta^2 values of ANOVA. Consequently, the correlation will be higher, in general, and require higher values for statistical significance, since there are greater degrees of freedom in ANOVA compared to correlational approaches (i.e., df = 3,55 compared to df = 1,48).

menstrual problems are solely with women who are figure skaters, gymnasts, and basketball players. The figure skaters report relatively high degrees of neurological problems and sleep loss. Gymnasts indicate a greater concern with increased use of coffee and tea, as well as digestive and weight problems. The two groups of gymnasts and figure skaters report relatively more problems and of longer duration compared to the other athletes.

Two different analyses were attempted in the hopes of identifying health and injury problems with specific life changes. Using Bramwell and colleagues [4] trichotomy, the life-change scores were divided into high, medium, and low and then compared to the incidence of health or injury problem. No significant findings were obtained, with the exception of increased nonprescription drug use for the high life-change group.

The second analysis was to compare positive and negative life-change events with respect to health and injury problems. Some researchers have suggested that negative events (such as death of a relative or divorce) should be more predictive of health problems than positive events. The authors reviewed each item where response variation allowed calculation of correlations, judging it positive, negative, or nonclassifiable (this latter category

Table 12.3 Average Frequency and Duration (in Days) of Health Problems
by Sport

| | Mean Number of Days | | | | |
Problem	Gymnastics	Figure Skating	Basket-ball	Biathalon	Race-walking
(sample size)	(10)	(4)	(6)	(19)	(18)
	Problem-Frequency (mean incidence)				
Eyes**	1.8	0	0.5	0.2	0.1
Menstrual***	2.5	7.0	1.8	0	0
Musculoskeletal (back)*	2.3	0	0.2	0.5	0.3
Neurological-dizziness**	0.9	4.3	0	0.3	0.1
Sleep loss***	2.5	11.0	3.8	1.2	1.9
Weight gain/loss**	2.5	1.0	0.7	0.2	0.8
	Problem-Duration (mean number of days)				
Headache*	3.6	2.3	0	0.9	1.6
Eyes**	3.3	0	0.8	0.2	0.1
Digestive**	12.0	35.0	3.3	3.4	1.3
Sleep loss*	2.6	35.0	1.8	7.6	4.3
Weight gain/loss***	20.0	0	0	0	6.8
Increased coffee/tea consumption**	24.0	1.8	2.3	0	0.2

Using one-way ANOVA, asterisks denote significant differences between sport activity.
*$p<.10$ **$p<.05$ ***$p<.01$

could be positive or negative depending on the person or situation).
Of these 40 items, 21 were consequently judged to be clearly
negative (e.g., major injury), 3 were judged positive (e.g., an out-
standing personal achievement award), and the remaining 16 were
nonclassifiable (e.g., changing to new school or team). The
correlations with the 25 HIPS items were then examined. A
chi-square comparison of the proportion of significant correlations (using alpha $p < .05$) showed a significant effect ($X^2 = 6.77$,
df $= 2, p < .02$).

Only in the case of the negative item group, however, did the
number of significant correlations exceed that which could be
expected on the basis of chance using an alpha level of .05. In brief,
the negative items do seem to be somewhat more associated with
health problems. The oversimplified classification system and the
small actual differences between the negative and positive groups of

items, however, precludes an unequivocal interpretation, especially since the trend was for "positive" items also to be in the direction of greater health problems.

National ranking as indicators of performance were not significantly related to life-change scores. However, regional rankings were strongly associated with life-change scores ($r = .693, p < .004$). This relationship was even stronger when regional ranking for the six months immediately prior to the HIPS survey were correlated with life changes for the six months immediately prior to the life-change survey, actually an interval of one year. In this case, 64% of the variation in performance rankings can be explained by the life-change scores ($r = .80; p < .001$). Unfortunately, regional data was available for only 13 athletes which requires this finding to be interpreted with considerable caution.

DISCUSSION

The current study demonstrates that the amount of life change is an important force in an individual's life which may influence the onset of injury, illness, as well as the quality of athletic performance. Athletes, especially those experiencing high life changes, which can lead to considerable anxiety regarding performance, end up actually experiencing problems. As would be expected, these individuals have several health problems which are commonly related to stress, such as headaches, digestive tract disturbance, anxiety, and substance use.

The increased use of nonprescribed medication is of particular interest. It may well be that these indivuduals who experience high degrees of change are so anxious that they are avoiding going to the appropriate health care practitioner. This self-medication can lead to more problems, and therefore, their health and performance deteriorates even more. Unfortunately the current research project did not identify which nonprescription medications are being used, but hopefully further research will provide us with that information.

The relationship of other physical problems, such as orthopedic injuries, to these life changes, is of particular interest. The common myth is that accidents occur as a natural process of a sport or are the physical hazards of a particular activity. This study, as well as research discussed earlier, suggests that one component of injury and illness is an environmental or psychological factor. It may be that our ability to concentrate and attend to our environment is diminished when we experience considerable life change. The consequence of this finding is that the behavioral component is potentially preventable.

The evidence for negative life events being more influential in the onset of health problems is partially substantiated. Unfortunately, the life events scales developed by Holmes and Bramwell does not possess a large enough number of clearly defined positive events to answer the question adequately. The Sarason Life Experience Survey may be a more sensitive instrument to determine the relative influence of positive and negative events. It may be an oversimplification to expect that merely a negative or positive perception of the event would account for a significant amount of the variance. The individual's coping ability may be another important variable and is being investigated on subsequent research.

The effects of life events and their relationship to regional performance ranking is suggestive that performance level deteriorates with the increasing life events within the regionally ranked athletes. Unfortunately the database for this section of the study was extremely small and therefore is speculative. The regional rankings of the less experienced and younger group of athletes did show the expected results.

An interesting finding with respect to the influence of the type of sport is that younger, developmental athletes tended to be more vulnerable to life stresses, as for example, the basketball team. This is somewhat of a contradiction to previously held opinions that older people are more susceptible to illness and injury as a result of accumulating life events. It may well be that the younger, developmental athlete has not yet learned the psychological coping skills or the psychological preparation skills to be as efficient or consistent as the elite athlete. As a consequence he or she may be more susceptible to stress-related problems as they relate to their sport. One of the authors (J. M.) notices this tendency with young athletes in his clinical work. The highly skilled and internationally competitive athletes have frequently prepared themselves in all aspects of their sport and therefore cope with change and seem to be at less risk. Also, it follows that their performance is more successful.

A potential outgrowth from the current findings is the concept of preventative psychological measures. Most athletes spend considerable time on the physical aspect of their sport; however, they train unsystematically toward psychological fitness. It may someday be possible through psychological preparation, stress management, and other psychological training strategies to reduce the psychological risk component and thereby to reduce the illness and injury rate and increase the athlete's overall performance. These are interesting speculations and further research should also be conducted in this area. It is hoped that athletes. coaches, and team physicians will begin to study and work with the psychological side of their sport to a greater extent.

ACKNOWLEDGMENTS

Funding for the project was provided in part by the U.S. Olympic Sports Medicine Program and Grant #14514, Psychiatry Education Branch, National Institutes of Mental Health.

REFERENCES

1. Rosenblum S. Psychologic factors in competitive failures in athletes. *American Journal of Sports Medicine*, 7(3), 198-200, 1979.
2. Green, B. A., Gabrielsen, M. A., Hall, W. J., and O'Heir, J. Analysis of Swimming pool accidents resulting in spinal cord injury. *Parapegia*, *18*, 20, 1980.
3. Holmes, T., and Rahe, R. The social readjustment rating scale. *Journal of Psychosomatic Research*, *11*, 213-218, 1967.
4. Bramwell, S., Masuda, M., Wagner, N., and Holmes, T. Psychosocial factors in athletic injuries: Development and application of the social and athletic readjustment scale (SARRS). *Journal of Human Stress*, *1*(2), 6-20, 1975.
5. Coddington, R., and Troxwell, J. The effects of emotional factors on football injury rates—A pilot study. *Journal of Human Stress*, *4*(6), 2-6, 1980.
6. Seese, M. *Life Stress and Athletic Injuries*. Unpublished Master's thesis, Kinesiology. University of Washington, 1981.
7. Sarason J. G., Johnson, J. H., and Siegel, J. M. Assessing the impact of life changes: Development of the life experiences survey. *Journal of Consulting and Clinical Psychology*, *46*(5), 932-946, 1978.
8. Christensen, J. Psychological variables mediating life changes and illness patterns among recently married, divorced, and widowed populations. Unpublished doctoral dissertation, Psychology. University of Nevada, 1980.

IV.
Physiology

CHAPTER **13**

Profiles of Elite Athletes: Physical and Physiological Characteristics

Nancy Kay Butts

INTRODUCTION

The athletes of today run and swim faster, throw further, and jump higher than their counterparts of the past. For example, in 1925 the high-jump record was 6′6″ and 4′11¾″ for men and women, respectively, compared to the current records of 7′9″ and 6′8″. The 1500-meter track records were 3:53.6 and 5:44.0 for men and women, respectively, in 1925 compared to the record times of 3:30.76 and 3:52.47 at the time of this writing. These are only a few examples of the improvements in athletic performances that have occurred over the past fifty years.

These improvements may be due to many factors such as nutrition, better training techniques, motivation, recognition, governmental support, selection, and other factors too numerous to mention. In recent years much attention has been given to those quantitative factors that may distinguish the elite athlete from their less successful counterparts. Although there are many components that may separate the elite athlete from other performers, the largest

The Elite Athlete, edited by N. K. Butts, T. T. Gushiken, and B. Zarins. Copyright © 1985 by Spectrum Publications, Inc.

amount of research data have been directed toward the areas of physique and/or body composition, cardiorespiratory capacity, and muscle fiber characteristics.

Before we enter into a discussion concerning these characteristics, the elite athlete must first be defined and/or identified. Who is the elite athlete? Generally, an athlete is defined as a person trained in exercise or games requiring strength, skill, etc., and the elite is defined as a group or part of a group regarded as the best, most powerful, etc. Taking these definitions literally, one can find elite athletes at any and all levels of competition (i.e., elementary school, junior high, etc.); however, most people think of the elite athlete as those individuals who are successful in national or international competition, such as the Olympics. These national and international athletes are the ones who are identified as elite within the context of this chapter. In the search of information relative to these elite athletes, only references which have clearly identified their subjects as succesful in national or international levels of competition will be labeled as elite. Other individuals who are trained and/or engage in specific sports or athletic events will be simply referred to as trained.

PHYSICAL CHARACTERISTICS

Introduction

One of the most common comparisons often made between athletes and nonathletes has dealt with physique. For example Lon Myers, who held the American record of 4:27.6 for the mile in 1882, was described by a contemporary as "never was a man more naturally cut out for running than L. E. Myers. He is narrow chested and next to no weight about the hips . . ." [1]. Although Myers, who at 5'7¾" was average in height, he weighed only 114 lbs. Considering the average male of today who stands 5'8" and weighs approximately 150 lbs, it is apparent that Myers did not have a typical physique.

Somatotypes

A common technique frequently used to compare the physiques of Olympic athletes has been somatotyping, which is simply a means of describing the degree of roundness (endomorphy), muscle mass (mesomorphy), and linearity (ectomorphy) of the body. Various researchers have extensively studied the various somatotypes of

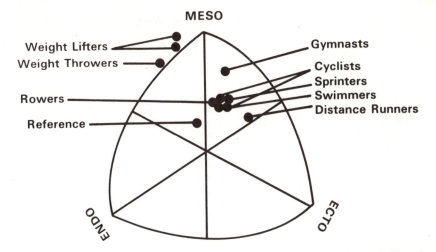

Figure 13.1. Mean somatoplots of males at 1960 [2], 1972 [3], and 1976 [4] Olympics.

participants of the 1960 [2], 1972 [3] and 1976 [4] Olympic games. An overview of somatotypes for selected male and female Olympic competitors are presented in Figures 13.1 and 13.2, respectively.

In general, these athletes, both male and female, tend to have a larger mesomorphic component (i.e., proportionately more muscle mass) and a smaller endomorphic component (i.e., proportionately

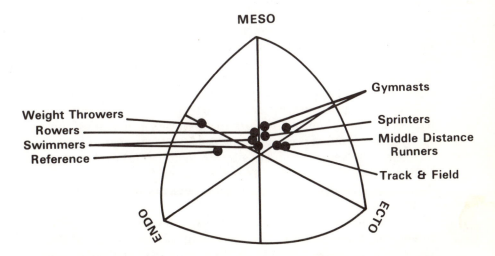

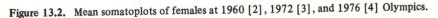

Figure 13.2. Mean somatoplots of females at 1960 [2], 1972 [3], and 1976 [4] Olympics.

Table 13.1. Heights and Weights of 10 of World's Best Male Marathoners

Name	Country	Age	Height	Weight	Marathon
Carlos Lopes	Por	36	168	57.3	2:07.11
Alberto Salazar	US	25	180	68.5	2:08.13
Rob deCastella	Aus	26	180	65.0	2:08.18
Toshiko Seko	Jap	27	165	53.2	2:08.38
Dick Beardsley	US	27	175	59.1	2:08.54
Takeshi Soh	Jap	30	178	58.2	2:08.55
Greg Meyer	US	27	178	65.0	2:09.01
Rodolfo Gomez	Mex	33	173	57.3	2:09.12
Juma Ikangaa	Tan	25	163	54.5	2:09.30
Armand Parmentier	Bel	29	175	66.4	2:09.57
Average		**28.5**	**173.5**	**60.5**	

Source: New Balance Marathon Times (pp. 8–9), Fall 1983 (with revisions).

less fat) when compared to the reference or average individual. It appears that the specific somatotypes of individual athletes are directly related to their sport. Obvious examples are the distance runners who tend to have a higher ectomorphy component compared to the higher mesomorphy component for weight lifters and throwers. For a comprehensive overview, the reader is directed to the works of Tanner [2], deGaray et al. [3] and Carter et al. [4].

Height and Weight

The most common assessment of physique simply involves height and weight measurements. Individual height and weights of 10 of the world's best male and female marathoners are presented in Tables 13.1 and 13.2 [5]. For comparison purposes, the average height and weight of Americans in their twenties are approximately 177 cm and 75.7 kg for males and 163 cm and 61 kg for females, respectively [6]. As a group, the male marathoner's average height is approximately 3.5 cm shorter and his weight 15 kg lower than the comparison male. The female runners also are lighter (10 kg), but they are slightly taller (3 cm) than the comparison female. As with the population in general, the heights and weights of these elite marathoners are quite variable.

Average heights and weight obtained for various other groups of female and male elite athletes are graphically presented in Figures 13.3 and 13.4, respectively. With the exception of volleyball players, rowers, and throwers, the majority of the male athletes are in the

Table 13.2. Heights and Weights of 10 of World's Best Female Marathoners

Name	Country	Age	Height	Weight	Marathon
Ingred Kristiansen	Nor	27	170	52.3	2:21.06
Joan Benoit	US	26	160	47.7	2:22.43
Grete Waitz	Nor	29	173	54.1	2:25.29
Allison Roe	NZ	27	175	59.1	2:25.29
Julie Brown	US	28	168	49.1	2:26.24
Charlotte Teske	WG	33	168	55.0	2:29.02
Mary O'Connor	NZ	28	155	43.2	2:28.20
Carey May	Ire	24	165	49.1	2:29.23
Jacqueline Gareau	Can	29	157	45.5	2:29.23
Nancy Conz	US	26	173	53.2	2:33.23
Average		**27.7**	**166.4**	**50.8**	

Source: New Balance Marathon Times (pp. 8-9), Fall, 1983 (with revisions).

middle or average range for height. In contrast, the height of the majority of the female athletes tend to be skewed to the taller end of the spectrum. The total body weights of the athletes, excluding the exceptionally tall groups (volleyball, throwers, and weight lifters), appear to be below that of the values reported for the comparison male and female of similar ages. Obviously there are individual exceptions within each of these groups since these values represent group means. The significance of the lower weights of the elite athlete is further discussed below.

Percent Body Fat

In recent years comparisons of the body fat of various athletes have replaced the simpler height and weight measures as a more definitive means of comparing the body composition of various groups of athletes. Percentage of body fat can be estimated using various prediction equations or measured via hydrostatic weighing. Although estimates of the percentage of body fat of elite athletes by prediction equations have been presented by numerous researchers, only values determined through hydrostatic weighing are presented in Figures 13.3 and 13.4.

With the exception of female middle-distance swimmers and throwers [7] and male throwers [8], these athletes have percentages body fat below the 15–17% and 25% generally reported for the average male and female respectively [9]. This observation is apparently consistent regardless of the caliber or the age of the athlete.

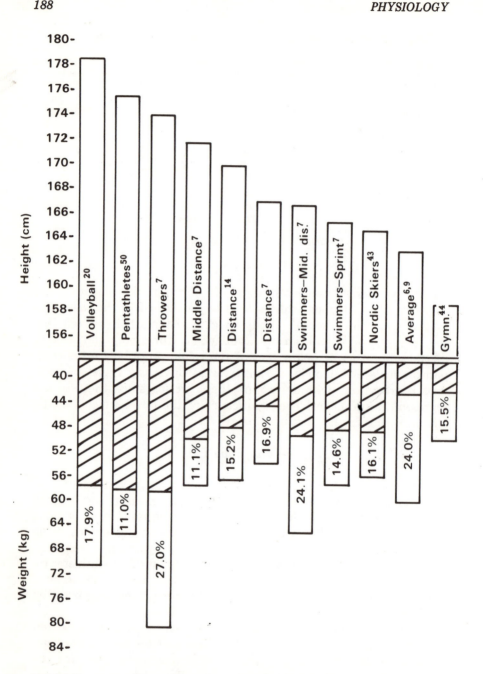

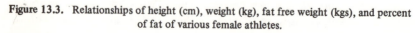

Figure 13.3. Relationships of height (cm), weight (kg), fat free weight (kgs), and percent of fat of various female athletes.

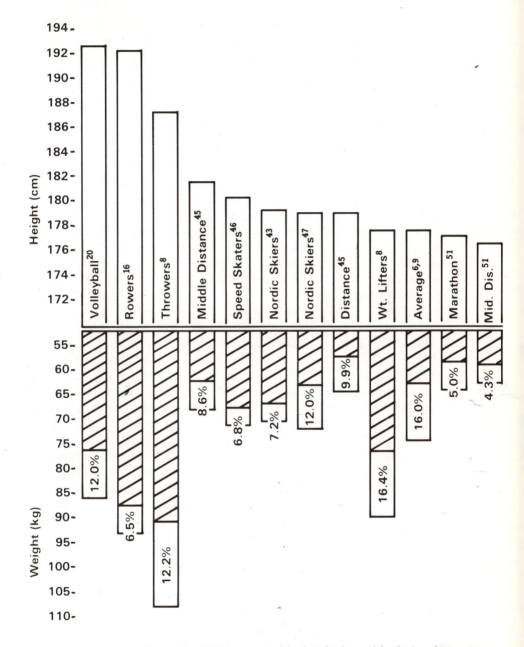

Figure 13.4.   Relationships of height (cm), weight (kg), fat free weight (kgs), and percent of fat of various male athletes.

For example, young (15.6 years) nonelite female cross-country runners' percentage body fat of 15.3% [10] is similar to the 15.2% reported for older (32.4 years) elite female distance runners [7]. Although the majority of elite athletes tend to have a lower percentage of body fat than the average individual, it appears that percentage body fat itself does not distinguish the elite athlete from their less successful counterparts.

When comparing the percentage body fat of various groups of athletes, regardless of sex, it becomes apparent that the lower body fats are found in those athletes who have to support and/or move their body mass during their performances (i.e., runners, gymnasts, etc.). The relatively higher values are found in those athletes whose body weight is supported (i.e., swimmers, rowers, etc.) or are involved in events which require applying a force to an object rather than to their body mass (i.e., discus, shot, etc.). In addition, the intensive training regimens which require higher caloric expenditures may, in turn, contribute to the relatively lower percentages body fat reported for those athletes.

To further clarify this, Malina et al. [11] investigated the fatness and fat patterning of 456 male and female athletes who participated in the 1976 Olympics. Based upon the results they concluded that "either regular physical activity, such as training for sport, is likely to affect one's overall fatness, that the amount of body fat influence proficiency in sport, or some combination of these" (p. 450).

Natural selection, however, may be the greatest factor influencing the body composition and structure of various elite athletes. It would be hard to imagine L. E. Myers at 5'7¾" and 114 lbs. becoming an elite shot putter. Assuming people tend to become interested in those sports or activities in which they can experience success and avoid those in which they cannot, one could speculate that a combination of self-selection, biomechanical factors, and energy requirements contribute to the similarities in body composition and structure of the elite within a given sport.

CARDIORESPIRATORY

Aerobic Power

Perhaps because of its relative ease of measurement and its apparent importance to the success of many activities, cardiorespiratory endurance or aerobic power ($\dot{V}O_2$ max) has been extensively reported for various groups of athletes and nonathletes. The cardiorespiratory characteristics of elite athletes are well documented, and

Table 13.3. $\dot{V}O_2$ max Values for Various Elite Male Athletes in
Last Ten Years

Sport	N	Age	$L \cdot min^{-1}$	$ml \cdot kg \cdot min^{-1}$	Ref.
Volleyball	8	26.1	4.80	56.1	20
Hockey	23	22.1	4.38	54.0	52
Hockey	13	22.5	4.75	61.5	26
Alpine Skier	12	21.8	5.03	66.6*	53
Alpine Skier	6	21.2	4.45	63.8	26
CC Skier	10	22.7	5.34	73.0	53
CC Skier	17	25.6	5.42	78.3	26
Rowers	25	22.8	5.63	62.7*	54
Rowers	14	25.8	5.89	63.0	16
Rowers	13	25.1	5.58	67.0	16
Rowers	21	—	6.60	73.5	17
Rowers	6	—	5.36	67.0	18
Middle Distance	42	21.7	4.73	68.9	45
Long Distance	34	22.8	4.96	76.9	45
Long Distance	12	24.6	4.63*	71.7	15
Long Distance	8	26.2	5.19	78.1	24
Long Distance	14	26.2	4.95	77.4	13

*Estimated from data
$L \cdot min^{-1}$ = absolute value of $V\dot{O}_2$ max
$ml \cdot kg \cdot min^{-1}$ = $\dot{V}O_2$ max relative to body weight

Tables 13.3 and 13.4 provide a brief summary of the average $\dot{V}O_2$ max values obtained for various groups of male and female elite athletes obtained within the last 10 years. In addition, some specific individual values of various elite athletes are presented in Table 13.5.

Table 13.4. $\dot{V}O_2$ max Values for Various Elite Female Athletes in
Last Ten Years

Sport	N	Age	$L \cdot min^{-1}$	$ml \cdot kg \cdot min^{-1}$	Ref.
Volleyball	14	21.6	3.57	50.6	20
Volleyball	9	24.4	2.77	44.2	55
Penathlete	6	22.2	3.55*	50.0	56
Penathlete	9	21.5	3.00	45.9	50
Alpine Skier	13	19.5	3.10	52.2*	53
CC Skier	10	20.2	3.44	61.5	53
Distance Runner	11	32.4	3.34	59.1	14
Distance Runner	14	20.0	3.43*	62.0	56

*Estimated from data
$L \cdot min^{-1}$ = absolute value of $V\dot{O}_2$ max
$ml \cdot kg \cdot min^{-1}$ = $\dot{V}O_2$ max relative to body weight

Table 13.5. $\dot{V}O_2$ max Values for Selected Individuals from Reference Cited in Text

Athlete	Sex	$L \cdot min^{-1}$	$ml \cdot kg \cdot min^{-1}$
Finnish Skier	M	6.50	93.0
Am. Skier	M	6.20	88.0
Prefontaine	M	5.60*	84.4
Scott	M	5.85	80.1
G. Meyer	M	—	80.0
Ryun	M	5.75	79.5
Benoit	F	3.77*	79.0
Finnish Skier	F	4.40	75.0
Snell	M	5.50	73.0
Shorter	M	4.37*	71.3
Clayton	M	—	69.7
Decker	F	—	67.0
DeMar (@49 yr.)	M	3.64	60.0

*Estimated from data
$L \cdot min^{-1}$ = absolute value of $\dot{V}O_2$ max
$ml \cdot kg \cdot min^{-1}$ = $\dot{V}O_2$ max relative to body weight

It has been suggested that to be successful in world competition, endurance athletes must have relatively high $\dot{V}O_2$ max values (i.e., greater than 70 $ml \cdot kg \cdot min^{-1}$ for males [12], but having a high $\dot{V}O_2$ max does not, in itself, predict success among elite athletes. It is interesting to note that Pollock et al. [21] found that, on the average, middle-distance runners had significantly higher $\dot{V}O_2$ max values (77.8 $ml \cdot kg \cdot min^{-1}$) than elite marathoners (74.1 $ml \cdot kg \cdot min^{-1}$). If $\dot{V}O_2$ max were the major factor influencing endurance performances, then the opposite result would have been expected. To further illustrate the fact that a high $\dot{V}O_2$ max is not the sole factor in successful distance running, Costill and associates [13] reported that Derek Clayton, who held the world marathon record for years, had a $\dot{V}O_2$ max of 69.7 $ml \cdot kg \cdot min^{-1}$ and Frank Shorter, another world-class marathoner, had a $\dot{V}O_2$ max of 71.3 $ml \cdot kg \cdot min^{-1}$. Recently the complete roster of the University of Wisconsin at La Crosse NCAA Division III men's (n = 44) and women's (n = 27) cross-country teams were tested. The men averaged 71.8 and the women 59.8 $ml \cdot kg \cdot min^{-1}$. Although these are high $\dot{V}O_2$ max values, and the men placed third and the women first in their respective national championships, these runners cannot be viewed as world class even though their $\dot{V}O_2$ maxs were comparable to elite women [14] and men [15] runners. A relatively high $\dot{V}O_2$ max may be necessary for successful endurance performance, but the previous examples illustrate that perhaps after a minimum level is reached, $\dot{V}O_2$ max itself may not be a discriminating factor in the performance of the elite endurance athlete.

While elite runners and cross-country skiers tend to have the highest $\dot{V}O_2$ max when expressed relative to body weight (ml·kg·min^{-1}), some of the highest absolute values (L·min^{-1}) have been consistently reported for elite oarsmen [16,17,18]. This is due, in part, to the differences in body mass reported earlier. Runners must support their body weights throughout the race while the water supports the oarsmen, thus size is not a disadvantage to them. It is interesting to note that although the $\dot{V}O_2$ max expressed relative to body weight for the most successful oarsmen [16,19] were similar to those of less successful oarsmen, their absolute $\dot{V}O_2$ max were significantly higher. Larsson and Forsberg [19] have suggested that even though a larger muscle mass might negatively influence resistance in the water, the potential metabolic and biomechanical benefits gained with the increase body size may well compensate for this increased resistance. The importance of absolute $\dot{V}O_2$ max values in these athletes was further emphasized recently when Tesch [18] suggested a minimum value of 4.9 L·min^{-1} is desired for success in 1,000-meter kayak racing.

Although the $\dot{V}O_2$ max values reported for other groups of elite athletes are higher than the values typically reported for the untrained, they fall below those commonly reported for endurance athletes. In activities such as volleyball, basketball, etc., factors other than cardiorespiratory endurance appear to be more related to success. Some of these factors may include anaerobic power, experience, training, skill, innate ability, selection, etc. Many of these factors are hard to assess quantitatively. Recently Puhl et al. [20] measured various physical and physiological characteristics of male and female volleyball players. They found little difference in the physiological variables between the elite and less skilled players and suggested that innate physical characteristics do not appear to discriminate between the elite and less skilled volleyball players. Rather they suggested that total time playing the game and self-selection may be the major discriminating factors.

Efficiency

Another factor to be considered is the individual's efficiency of movement, especially in running events. Pollock et al. [21] pointed out that even though both Clayton's and Shorter's $\dot{V}O_2$ max were not exceptionally high, both individuals were extremely economical runners. This simply means that at a given pace their energy cost was less. Although Costill et al. [22] suggested that submaximal oxygen uptake is not related to performance, Conley and Krahenbuhl [15] found that 65% of the variation observed in the performance of running a 10,000-meter race was related to the running economy within a group of highly trained runners. In a 1984 study [23], the running economy of Steve Scott was compared to that of Jim Ryun. Both Ryun and Scott had similar $\dot{V}O_2$ max of 79.5 and 80.1 ml·kg· min^{-1}, respectively; however, during a standard submaximal pace Ryun's oxygen consumption was 49 compared to 45.9 ml·kg·min^{-1} for Scott. They concluded that "the essential difference between Scott and the former American record holder in the mile, Jim Ryun, appeared to be running economy, which may have allowed Scott to perform a standard workload at a smaller percentage of his maximal aerobic capacity" (p. 106).

Relative Intensity

Related to both $\dot{V}O_2$ max and efficiency is the ability of the individual to utilize a larger fraction of his aerobic capacity during competition. Even though a person may have a relatively low $\dot{V}O_2$ max, he may be able to work at a higher percentage of this value before lactate accumulates, thus negating the actual difference in maximal values. Theoretically, if two runners had similar running efficiencies and similar $\dot{V}O_2$ maxs, but one could run at a higher relative intensity (% $\dot{V}O_2$ max) without significant lactate formation, that individual should be more successful. The following example illustrates this point. If runner A had a $\dot{V}O_2$ max of 80 ml·kg·min^{-1} and could run at 75% and runner B, whose $\dot{V}O_2$ max was 70 ml·kg· min^{-1}, could run at 85%, they both would be expending approximately 60 ml·kg·min^{-1}. However, if runner B was a more efficient runner than A, theoretically his 60 ml·kg·min^{-1} expenditure could represent a faster pace. Basically it appears that the most successful endurance athlete will be the one who has the highest $\dot{V}O_2$ max, the highest running efficiency, and can run at the highest relative intensity.

MUSCLE FIBER CHARACTERISTICS

Introduction

Only in the last twenty-five years has the muscle biopsy technique been employed to identify the muscle fiber types of individuals and/or athletes. Since this technique is relatively new and rather complex, the information obtained has been somewhat limited to relatively few male and even fewer female athletes. In addition, the majority of the research has been restricted to the vastus lateralis, gastrocnemius, and deltoid muscles. The general information elicited from these biopsy studies has focused on the determination of the percentage of slow twitch (ST) and fast twitch (FT) fibers and their relative sizes. The ST or Type I fiber is characterized as having a high oxidative potential and is viewed as important for endurance-oriented events. In contrast, FT or Type II fibers are those associated with strength and/or power events and characterized as having high glycolytic potential.

Distribution

Do the muscles of the elite athlete differ from others in terms of the percentage and size of ST and FT fibers? Before this question can be addressed, a baseline or reference point for the nonathlete has to be identified.

In 1973, a comprehensive study of the size and distribution of 36 different human muscles obtained from autopsies of six nonathlete males subjects, ranging from 17 to 30 years of age, was presented in a series of articles [24,25]. All samples were removed from one side of the body within 24 hours of the subject's sudden death, and fiber types were identified via myofibrillar ATPase preparations with no differentiation between Type IIa and Type IIb fibers. The mean proportion of the ST and FT fibers are presented in Table 13.6. Since the researchers observed such extreme variability in the percentages of ST and FT fibers among subjects and muscles, they statistically calculated the percentage of ST and FT for each muscle site expected to fall within the 95% confidence limits. These values are also included in Table 13.6. As can be seen, there was wide variation in the relative percentage of ST and FT fibers between the various muscles and between individuals.

Returning to the original question, is there a difference in the proportion of ST and FT fibers when the untrained or average individual is compared to the trained and elite athlete? Assuming the values presented by Johnson et al. [24] are indicative of the percentage of ST and FT fibers in the average male, then an attempt at comparing them to the athletes' values can be undertaken. It should be noted, however, that exact comparisons between various studies are limited since many authors have not provided specific details regarding the exact site or depths of their biopsy procedures.

Table 13.6. Distribution of Muscle Fibers in Nonathletic Men

Muscle	%ST	%FT	95% range for %ST
Deltoid			
(superficial)	53.3	46.7	43.4–63.2
(deep)	61.0	39.0	46.2–75.7
Gastrocnemius			
(lat. head sup.)	43.5	56.5	37.4–49.6
(lat. head deep)	50.3	49.7	43.3–52.2
(medial head)	50.8	49.2	45.6–56.0
Vastus lateralis			
(superficial)	37.8	62.2	19.6–45.8
(deep)	46.9	53.1	37.5–56.2

Source: Adapted from Johnson, M. A., Polgar, J., Weightman, D., and Appleton, D. "Data on the distribution of fibre types in thirty-six human muscle." In *J. Neurol. Sci., 18*, 111–129, 1973.
ST = slow twitch; FT = fast twitch

Vastus Lateralis. Because of its location and importance in many athletic activities, the vastus lateralis has been extensively studied (Figure 13.5). Johnson et al. [24] estimated that 95% of the population's percentage of ST fibers should fall between 19.6 to 45.8% and 37.5 to 56.2% at the surface and deep levels, respectively. The majority of values reported for untrained males [19,26,27,28, 29,30] fall within these ranges. One study [31], however, reported a value of 57.7% for the ST fibers of the vastus lateralis in 19 untrained subjects which falls just outside the expected rance. The percentage of ST fibers reported for active and/or trained males also have been reported within these ranges [30,31,32,33]. Exceptions are trained endurance runners [32] and some athletes reported by Gollnick and associates [27]. It is hard to categorize many of these athletes as athletes as elite or just trained since no specific information was given on actual performances in many of these studies.

Some researchers have also reported the percentage of ST fibers in the vastus lateralis of elite athletes to fall within this range. For example, paddlers [32], sprinters/jumpers [26,29], power events [26], and cyclists [31] all had percentages of ST fibers within this range. This might be expected since these elite athletes compete in events which either do not require a large contribution from the vastus lateralis or are characterized as power events which require more short, high intensity energy expenditures which would not necessitate as much input from ST fibers.

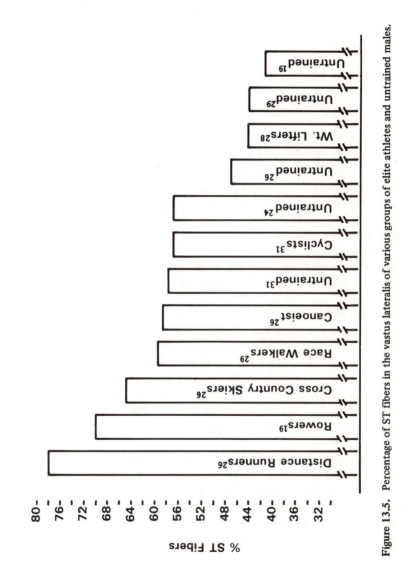

Figure 13.5. Percentage of ST fibers in the vastus lateralis of various groups of elite athletes and untrained males.

In contrast, when comparing the percent of ST fibers in the vastus lateralis of elite athletes whose events require high levels of endurance and/or major involvement of the vastus lateralis, the values generally fall outside the 95% range. These elite athletes have included race walkers [29], rowers [19], long-distance runners [26], speed skaters [26], and skiers [26].

Gastrocnemius. Not as clear of a pattern emerges when the percentage of ST fibers of the lateral head of the gastrocnemius are compared in various groups (Figure 13.6). The 95% range, accounting for the depth of the sample, has been reported to be between 37.4 and 57.2% ST [24] in the gastrocnemius. Although Coyle and colleagues' [34] values for untrained males fall within this range, the 57.7% reported for untrained males by Costill et al. [13] and Fink et al. [35] are slightly higher.

Clarkson et al. [32] endurance-trained athletes' percentage of ST fibers in the gastrocnemius fell into this range as did the values reported on good middle-distance runners. Other endurance trained athletes [13,32,35] were found to have higher percentages of ST fibers. A higher percentage of ST fibers was also found in the elite runners reported by both Costill et al. [13] and Fink et al. [35]. In fact, these authors reported values as high as 92, 96, and 98% ST in the gastrocnemius of selected elite runners. In contrast, elite shot putters had values in the normal range [34]. These results suggest the possibility that the percentage of ST fibers in the gastrocnemius may be even more related to endurance running success than the percentage of ST fibers in the vastus lateralis. This relationship may manifest itself more definitively when as many studies have been completed on the gastrocnemius of elite athletes as have been reported for the vastus lateralis.

Deltoid. Relatively few researchers have investigated the fiber types of the arm muscles. Gollnick et al. [27] reported percentage of ST fibers in the deltoid of various athletes and nonathletes to range from a low of 46.0% in untrained males to a high of 74.3% in five swimmers. Larsson and Forsberg [19] also reported 74.0% ST fibers in the deltoid of elite rowers. Although these athletes' values appear to be rather high, they fall within the 95% confidence range calculated for the average male [24]. At this time it is not clear if the fiber type distribution of ST in the deltoid supports the concept that the elite athletes whose performances require arm endurance (i.e., swimmers, rowers, paddlers, etc.) have a higher percentage of

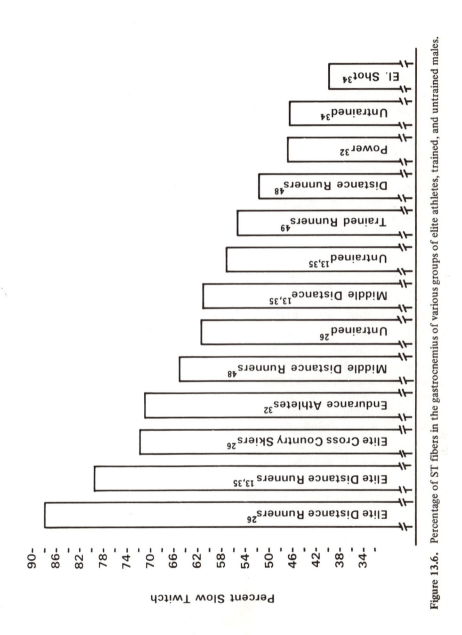

Figure 13.6. Percentage of ST fibers in the gastrocnemius of various groups of elite athletes, trained, and untrained males.

ST muscle fibers in their deltoids than the typical male or trained athlete.

On the basis of information currently presented in the literature, it appears that world-class or elite athletes may have a distribution of fiber types that distinguishes them from the population in general and also from their less successful counterparts. Perhaps this difference is best demonstrated by the percentage of ST fibers found in the gastrocnemius of the elite runners. It is generally accepted that the distribution of fibers is genetically determined [36] although function obviously plays a part [37]. Again it appears that selection of the sport may be a function of the success and/or failure of the individual at an early stage of participation. This early success may be dependent in part upon the distribution of fiber types in that individual which provides him/her with the natural element required for success.

Size

Even with the methodological problems involved, it is relatively simpler to compare the proportion or distribution of ST and FT fibers from study to study than it is to compare the size or cross-sectional area of the ST and FT fibers obtained by various researchers. Not only is the depth and exact location of the biopsy important, but the degree of fiber shortening at the time of the actual sampling can greatly influence the quantitative values obtained. In addition, some researchers have reported their data in diameters (μm) while others use the cross-sectional area (μ^2), thus making it difficult to make meaningful comparisons of actual values.

In an overview of muscle fiber composition, Saltin et al. [38] indicated that, in general, males have larger FT fibers than ST, but they did not indicate whether or not these differences were statistically significant. In 1973, Polgar et al. [25] found FT fibers to be larger than ST fibers in 44 of 50 muscle sites in average males. Although the FT fibers were larger than the ST in the vastus lateralis, gastrocnemius, and deltoid (see Table 13.7), these size differences were not found to be statistically significant in the average male. These results, indicating the size of the ST and FT fibers within a muscle are similar in the untrained or reference man, have been supported by others [13,28,30,34,35]. Thus, it appears that in the untrained, the size of the individual muscle fibers within a specific muscle are rather consistent regardless of whether they are identified as ST or FT fibers.

Table 13.7. Diameters of Muscle Fibers

Muscle	Diameters ST	FT
Deltoid		
(superficial)	51.6	58.6
(deep)	49.1	52.1
Gastrocnemius		
(lat. head sup.)	48.3	50.5
(lat. head deep)	48.4	50.5
(medial head)	65.0	66.0
Vastus lateralis		
(superficial)	63.1	63.2
(deep)	64.6	63.7

Source: Adapted from Polgar, J., Johnson, M. A., Weightman, D., and Appleton, D. "Data from fibre size of thirty-six human muscles." In *J. Neurol. Sci., 19,* 307–318, 1973.

When comparing the untrained individuals, the majority of studies have indicated that overall the trained individual has larger fibers, both ST and FT, than the untrained [13,27,31,34]. Is there, however, a difference in the size of the ST and FT fibers within the various muscles of athletes trained in various activities? In active runners [33] it was found that the FT fibers of the vastus lateralis were larger than the ST; however, Prince et al. [30] and Clarkson et al. [32] reported no difference in the ST and FT fiber size of the vastus lateralis in their trained runners. Likewise, in elite runners, Edstrom and Ekblom [28] did not find a difference in the size of the ST and FT fiber. Costill et al. [13] did not find good middle-distance runners to have a significant size difference in the gastrocnemius, but their elite runners had significantly larger ST than FT fibers. While endurance training appears to enhance the size of both the ST and FT fibers, the elite runners may have the capacity to enlarge their ST fibers to a greater degree than nonelite runners.

In contrast, larger FT than ST fibers have been reported in the vastus lateralis [30,32] and gastrocnemius [32] of trained weight lifters and in the vastus lateralis of elite lifters [28]. One study, however, found no difference in the fiber sizes of the ST and FT fibers of the gastrocnemius of elite shot putters [34].

Table 13.8. Statistical Comparisons of the Size of ST and FT Fibers in the Vastus Lateralis of Various Groups

Group	Size	Significance	Reference
Untrained	FT = ST	n.s.	30
	FT = ST	n.s.	28
	FT = ST	n.s.	25
Runners	FT = ST	n.s.	32
	FT = ST	n.s.	30
	FT = ST	n.s.	28
Weight Lifters	FT > ST	0.01	32
	FT > ST	0.005	30
Elite Weight Lifters	FT > ST	0.005	28

Many of the studies cited previously have indicated size differences between ST and FT fibers of various groups, but few indicated whether or not these differences were statistically significant. Those studies which included statistical data are summarized in Tables 13.8 and 13.9. On the basis of this statistical information, it appears that trained runners have larger muscle fibers, both ST and FT, than the untrained, but there is no significant difference between the size of their ST and FT fibers. The majority of information also indicates that many athletes, both trained and elite, who are engaged in weight lifting have significantly larger FT than ST fibers in their vastus lateralis and gastrocnemius. In contrast, significantly larger ST than FT fibers were found in the gastrocnemius of elite distance runners.

Table 13.9. Statistical Comparison of the Size of ST and FT Fibers in the Gastrocnemius of Various Groups

Group	Size	Significance	Reference
Untrained	FT = ST	n.s.	38
	FT = ST	n.s.	13,35
	FT = ST	n.s.	34
Middle Distance	FT = ST	n.s.	13,35
Weight Lifters	FT > ST	0.05	32
Elite			
Shot Putters	FT = ST	n.s.	34
Distance Runners	FT < ST	0.05	13,35

Only recently has definitive information been available on elite body builders. Tesch and Larsson [39] reported no difference in the ST and FT fiber size of three elite body builders in either the vastus lateralis or deltoid muscles, but the percentage of ST fibers was greater than the FT. Similar findings were reported in the triceps of seven elite power-lifters and body builders [40]. Tesch and Larsson [39] suggested that the training programs of competitive body builders may be increasing their musclar endurance as much, if not more, than strength, thus the ST fibers may be more important for success in body building. Both researchers [39,40] speculate that perhaps these body builders had a greater total number of muscle fibers initially that enable them to develop into world-class body builders.

In recent years, the single muscle biopsy technique employed in the above studies and the resulting interpretations have been questioned. Some of the researchers who have been most productive in the area of muscle study are encouraging restraint in using muscle biopsy information and have suggested "that the results of a single biopsy may not be conclusive" [41, p. 52]. In the early 1970s, the extreme variability of fiber distribution within a given muscle was reported [24] as well as the difference in the relative size of the fibers of various depths [25]. Recently Lexell et al. [42] again emphasized these findings. Through multiple sampling of the vastus lateralis, they clearly found a systematic difference in the distribution of fiber types within a muscle (i.e., increased depth resulted in a gradual increase in the percent of ST fibers). In addition, they found large variations between adjacent samples and thus concluded that fiber type distribution within the vastus lateralis is not randomly distributed.

Results of such studies, therefore, may limit the interpretations of the single muscle biopsy techniques employed by most investigators. However, even taking into account the nonrandomization of the distribution of the fibers within a muscle, some consistent patterns still surface. For example, elite distance runners appear to have an extremely high percentage of ST fibers in their leg muscles, especially the gastrocnemius. The elite runners also appear to have larger ST than FT fibers while the opposite appears in the muscle of elite power athletes. Furthermore, limited information suggests successful body builders may have a higher percentage of ST fibers with no size differentiation between their ST and FT fibers.

CONCLUSION

In order to truly ascertain those physical and physiological characteristics that may discriminate the elite from the less successful athlete, longitudinal data need to be collected on a large group of individuals over many years. This procedure may be possible in those countries which attempt to identify potential athletes at an early age and provide special schools and training programs for them. This approach, however, seems unlikely to occur within our present sports structure in the United States. The data currently being obtained at the Olympic Training Centers are a beginning, but at best, it will provide only generalized information on athletes after the selection process has occurred.

REFERENCES

1. Willis, J. D., and Wettan, R. G. L. E. Myers, "World's greatest runner." *J. Sport History, 2*(2), 95, 1975.
2. Tanner, J. M. *The physique of the Olympic athlete.* London, England: George Allen and Unwin Ltd., 1964.
3. deGaray, A. L., Levine, L., and Carter, J. E. L. *Genetic and anthropological studies of Olympic athletes.* New York: Academic Press, 1974.
4. Carter, J. E. L., Aubry, S. P., and Sleet, D. A. Somatotypes of Montreal Olympic athletes. *Med. Sci. Sports, 16*, 53-80, 1982.
5. *New balance marathon times.* 8-9, Fall, 1983.
6. U.S. Bureau of the Census. *Statistical abstract of the United States: 1982-83* (103 edition). Washington, DC: 1982.
7. Wilmore, J. H., Brown, C. H., and Davis, J. A. Body physique and composition of the female distance runner. *Ann. New York Acad., 301*, 764-776, 1977.
8. Fahey, T., Akka, L., and Rolph, R. Body composition and $\dot{V}O_2$ max of exceptional weight-trained athletes. *J. Appl. Physiol., 39*, 559-561, 1975.
9. Fox, E. L., and Mathews, D. K. *The physiological basis of physical education and athletes.* New York: Saunders College Publishing (p. 532), 1981.
10. Butts, N. K. Physiological profiles of high school female cross country runners. *Res. Quart. Exer. Sport, 53*(1), 8-14, 1982.
11. Malina, R. M., Mueller, W. H., Bouchard, C., Shoup, R. F., and Lariviere, G. Fatness and fat patterning among athletes at the Montreal Olympic games, 1976. *Med. Sci. Sports Exer., 14*(6), 445-452, 1982.
12. Pollock, M. L. Submaximal and maximal working capacity of elite distance runners cardiorespiratory aspects. *Ann. New York Acad. Sci., 301*, 310-322, 1977.

13. Costill, D. L., Fink, W. J., and Pollock, M. L. Muscle fiber composition and enzyme activities of elite distance runners. *Med. Sci. Sports*, *8*(2), 96-100, 1976.
14. Wilmore, J. H., and Brown, C. H. Physiological profiles of women runners. *Med. Sci. Sports*, *6*(3), 178-181, 1974.
15. Conley, D. L., and Krahenbuhl, G. S. Running economy and distance running performance of highly trained athletes. *Med. Sci. Sports Exer.*, *12*(5), 357-360, 1980.
16. Secher, N. H., Vaage, O., Jensen, K., and Jackson, R. C. Maximal aerobic power in oarsmen. *Eur. J. Appl. Physiol.*, *51*, 155-162, 1983.
17. Clark, J. M., Hagerman, F. C., and Gelfand, R. Breathing patterns during submaximal and maximal exercise in elite oarsmen. *J. Appl. Physio.*, *55*(2), 440-446, 1983.
18. Tesch, P. A. Physiological characteristics of elite Kayak paddlers. *Can. J. Appl. Sport Sci.*, *8*(2), 87-91, 1983.
19. Larsson, L., and Forsberg, A. Morphological muscle characteristics in rowers. *Can. J. Appl. Sport Sci.*, *5*(4), 239-244, 1980.
20. Puhl, J., Case, S., Fleck, S., and VanHandel, P. Physical and physiological characteristics of elite volleyball players. *Res. Quart. Exer. Sport*, *53*(3), 257-262, 1982.
21. Pollock, M. L., Jackson, A. S., and Pate, R. R. Discriminant analysis of physiological differences between good and elite distance runners. *Res. Quart. Exer. Sport*, *51*(3), 521-532, 1980.
22. Costill, D. L., Thomason, H., and Roberts, E. Fractional utilization of the aerobic capacity during distance running. *Med. Sci. Sports*, *5*(4), 248-252, 1973.
23. Conley, D. L., Krahenbuhl, G. S., Burkett, L. N., and Millar, A. L. Following Steve Scott: Physiological changes accompanying training. *Physician Sportsmed.*, *12*(1), 103-106, 1984.
24. Johnson, M. A., Polgar, J., Weightman, D., and Appleton, D. Data on the distribution of fibre types in thirty-six human muscles. *J. Neurol. Sci.*, *18*, 111-129, 1973.
25. Polgar, J., Johnson, M. A., Weightman, D., and Appleton, D. Data of fibre size in thirty-six human muscles. *J. Neurol. Sci.*, *19*, 307-318, 1973.
26. Rusko, H., Havu, M., and Karvinen, E. Aerobic performance capacity in athletes. *Eur. J. Appl. Physiol.*, *38*, 151-159, 1978.
27. Gollnick, P. D., Armstrong, R. B. Saltin, B., Saubert, IV, C. W., Sembrowich, W. L., and Shepherd, R. E. Effect of training on enzyme activity and fiber composition of human skeletal muscle. *J. Appl. Physiol.*, *34*(1), 107-111, 1973.
28. Edstrom, L., and Ekblom, B. Differences in sizes of red and white muscle fibres in vastus lateralis of musculus quadriceps femoris of normal individuals and athletes: Relation to physical performance. *Scand. J. Clin. Invest.*, *30*, 175-181, 1972.
29. Thorstensson, A., Larsson, L., Tesch, P., and Karlsson, J. Muscle strength and fiber composition in athletes and sedentary men. *Med. Sci. Sports*, *91*(1), 26-30, 1972.

30. Prince, F. P., Hikida, R. S., and Hagerman, F. C. Human muscle fiber types in power lifters, distance runners and untrained subjects. *Eur. J. Physiol.*, *363*, 19-26, 1976.

31. Burke, E. R., Cerny, F., Costill, D., and Fink, W. Characteristics of skeletal muscle in competitive cyclists. *Med. Sci. Sports*, *9*(2), 109-112, 1977.

32. Clarkson, P. M., Kroll, W., and McBride, T. C. Maximal isometric strength and fiber type composition in power and endurance athletes. *Eur. J. Appl. Physiol.*, *44*, 35-42, 1980.

33. Ivy, J. L., Costill, D. L., and Maxwell, B. D. Skeletal muscle determinants of maximal aerobic power in man. *Eur. J. Appl. Physiol.*, *44*, 1-8, 1980.

34. Coyle, E. F., Bell, S., Costill, D. L., and Fink, W. J. Skeletal muscle fiber characteristics of world class shot-putters. *Res. Quart.*, *49*(3), 278-284, 1978.

35. Fink, W. J., Costill, D. L., and Pollock, M. L. Submaximal and maximal working capacity of elite distance runners. Muscle fiber composition and enzyme activities. *Ann. New York Acad. Sci.*, *301*, 323-327, 1977.

36. Komi, P. V., Viitasalo, J. H., Havu, M., Thorstensson, Sjodin, B. and Karlsson, J. Skeletal muscle fibres and muscle enzyme activities in mono-zygous and dizygous twins of both sexes. *Acta Physiol. Scand.*, *100*, 385-392, 1977.

37. Fugi-Meyer, A. R., Eriksson, A., Sjostrom, M., and Soderstrom, G. Is muscle structure influenced by genetical or functional factors? *Acta Physiol. Scand.*, *114*, 277-281, 1982.

38. Saltin, B., Henriksson, J., Nygaard, E., and Andersen, P. Fiber types and metabolic potentials of skeletal muscles in sedentary man and endurance runners. *Ann. New York Acad. Sci.*, *301*, 3-29, 1977.

39. Tesch, P. A., and Larsson, L. Muscle hypertrophy in bodybuilders. *Eur. J. Appl. Physiol.*, *49*, 301-306, 1982.

40. MacDougall, J. D., Sale, D. G., Elder, G. C. B., and Sutton, J. R. Muscle ultrastructural characteristics of elite powerlifters and bodybuilders. *Eur. J. Appl. Physiol.*, *48*, 117-126, 1982.

41. Gollnick, P. D., Hermansen, L., and Salten, B. The muscle biopsy: Still a research tool. *Physician Sportsmed.* 8(1), 50-52, 1982.

42. Lexell, J., Henriksson-Larsen, K., and Sjostrom, M. Distribution of different fibre types in human skeletal muscles. *Acta Physiol. Scand.*, *117*, 115-122, 1983.

43. Sinning, W. E., Cunningham, L. N., Racaniello, P., and Sholes, J. L. Body composition and somatotype of male and female nordic skiers. *Res. Quart.*, *48*(4), 741-749, 1977.

44. Sinning, W. E., and Lindberg, G. D. Physical characteristics of college age women gymnasts. *Res. Quart.*, *43*(2), 226-234, 1972.

45. Boileau, R. A., Mayhew, J. L., Riner, W. F., and Lussier, L. Physiological characteristics of elite middle and long distance runners. *Can. Appl. Sport Sci.*, *7*(3), 167-172, 1982.

46. Pollock, M. L., Foster, C., Anholm, J., Hare, J., Farrell, P., Maksud, M., and Jackson, A. S. Body composition of Olympic speed skating candidates. *Res. Quart. Exer. Sport*, *53*(2), 150-155.

47. Hanson, J. S. Decline of physiologic training effects during the competitive season in members of the U.S. Nordic ski team. *Med. Sci. Sports, 1*(3), 213-216, 1975.
48. Taunton, J. E., Maron, H., and Wilkinson, J. G. Anaerobic performance in middle and long distance runners. *Can. J. Appl. Sport Sci., 6*(3), 109-113, 1981.
49. Foster, C., Costill, D. L., Daniels, J. T., and Fink, W. J. Skeletal muscle enzyme activity, fiber composition and $\dot{V}O_2$ max in relation to distance running performance. *Eur. J. Appl. Physiol. 39*, 73-80, 1978.
50. Krahenbuhl, G. S., Wells, C. L., Brown, C. H., and Ward, P. E. Characteristics of national and world class female pentathletes. *Med. Sci. Sports Exer. 11*(1), 20-23, 1979.
51. Pollock, M. L., Gettman, L. R., Jackson, A., Ayres, J., Ward, A., and Linnerud, A. C. Body composition of elite class distance runners. *Ann. New York Acad. Sci., 301*, 361-370, 1977.
52. Smith, D. J., Wenger, H. A., Quinney, H. A. Sexsmith, J. R., and Steadward, R. D. Physiological profiles of the Canadian Olympic hockey team (1980). *Can. J. Appl. Sport Sci., 7*(2):142-146, 1982.
53. Haymes, E. M., and Dickson, A. L. Characteristics of elite male and female ski racers. *Med. Sci. Sports Exer., 12*(3), 153-158, 1980.
54. Mickelson, T. C., and Hagerman, F. C. Anaerobic threshold measurements of elite oarsmen. *Med. Sci. Sports Exer., 14*(6), 440-444, 1982.
55. Spence, D. W., Disch, J. G., Fred, H. L., and Coleman, A. E. Descriptive profiles of highly skilled women volleyball players. *Med. Sci. Sports Exer., 12*(4), 229-302, 1980.
56. Gregor, R. J., Edgerton, V. R., Rozenek, R., and Castleman, K. R. Skeletal muscle properties and performance in elite female track athletes. *Eur. J. Appl. Physiol., 47*, 355-364, 1981.

CHAPTER **14**

Iron Status and Training

Jackie L. Puhl, Peter J. Van Handel, Luther L. Williams,
Patrick W. Bradley, and Sandra J. Harms

Cellular metabolism provides the mechanism for using oxygen coupled with the breakdown of food substances to supply adenosine triphosphate (ATP). ATP is the universal energy source for cell functions, including muscle contraction.

Iron plays an essential role in two of these three processes. Almost all (98%) of the oxygen transported in the blood is carried by hemoglobin (Hb) in red-blood cells (RBCs). Hemoglobin contains iron. Oxygen utilization (cellular respiration) includes a series of chemical reactions involving cytochromes in the electron transport chain. These cytochromes contain iron. In addition, myoglobin binds oxygen for "storage" in cells and helps transport oxygen across the cells to sites of utilization. Myoglobin also contains iron. Other iron-containing compounds are important in cellular respiration and include catalase, peroxidase, NADH, succinate, aldehyde, and alpha-glycerophosphate dehydrogenases, and xanthine oxidase [1]. Because of the involvement of iron in the transportation and use of oxygen, the iron status of the athlete could have implications for performance at either the circulatory level or at the level of cellular metabolism.

The Elite Athlete, edited by N. K. Butts, T. T. Gushiken, and B. Zarins. Copyright © 1985 by Spectrum Publications, Inc.

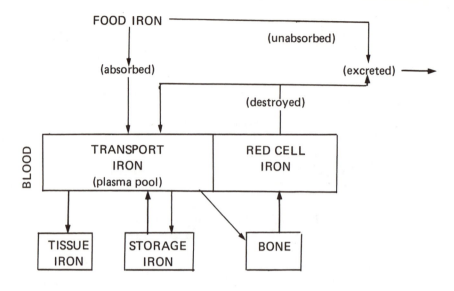

Figure 14.1. Iron metabolism.

BODY IRON STATUS

Factors involved in iron balance and iron deficiency and its assessment are discussed in the following sections. A general schema for iron metabolism is depicted in Figure 14.1.

Iron Balance

Adequate iron must be available for formation of hemoglobin (oxygen transport) and for muscle cell substances involved in oxygen utilization (metabolism). Iron availability depends on the balance between iron intake (absorption) and iron losses. An overview of iron balance is depicted in Figure 14.2. Average values for iron intake, absorption, and losses for men and women are shown in Table 14.1. The body iron content represents the results of the body's attempts to maintain iron balance. Average values for body iron holdings are shown in Table 14.2.

Iron Absorption

How much iron do we absorb from our dietary intake? Absorption is regulated by the amount of iron stored in the body. When

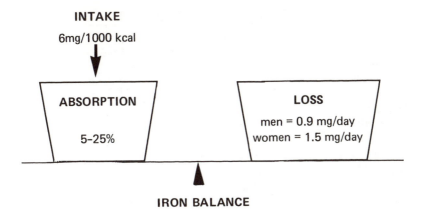

Figure 14.2. Iron balance.

iron stores are low, iron absorption increases; when stores are high, absorption decreases. Normally, about 5 to 15% of the dietary intake is absorbed [4,5]. In iron-depleted individuals, dietary iron absorption increases to about 10 to 20% [4,6,7,8,] with a maximum absorption rate of about 25% of the iron intake [2,8]. Recommendations for food iron intake usually assume about a 10% absorption rate [9]. Based on the wide individual variability of iron absorption, this assumption could be quite misleading.

Table 14.1. Average Iron Intake/Absorption and Losses

Iron Intake/Absorption (mg/day)[a]	Men	Women
RDA	10	18
Actual Intake	16	11
Absorption	0.9 (6%)	1.3 (12%)
Iron Depleted	10–20%	
Maximum Absorption	25%	

Iron Losses (mg/day)[b]	Men	Nonpregnant Women of Child-Bearing Age
GI Tract	0.6	Slightly < 0.6
Skin	0.2	Slightly < 0.2
Urine & Sweat	0.1	Slightly < 0.1
Menstruation	—	0.5
Total	0.9	1.4

a = from Munro, H. N. [2].
b = compiled from selected references listed in this chapter.

Table 14.2.   Body Iron Holdings

	Men (70 kg)		Women (57 kg)	%	
Red Cell Iron					
hemoglobin	2500*	2100	1750	67*	65
Transport Iron					
transferrin	3*	—	—	0.1*	
Storage Iron					
ferritin and hemosiderin	1000*	1000	400	27*	20
Other Iron		350			
myoglobin	130*			3.5*	
enzymes	8			0.2*	
miscible iron pool	80			2.2*	
Total	**3721**	**3450**	**2450**		

* = values from Fairbanks, V. F., et al. [3] ; other values from Munro, H. N. [2] .

The form in which the iron is ingested (heme or non-heme iron) modifies absorption. Heme iron constitutes about 50 to 60% of the iron in beef, lamb, and chicken and about 30 to 40% of the iron in fish, liver, and pork [10]. Heme iron appears to be absorbed at rates from 15 to 35% when iron stores range from 1000-0 mg iron [6]. For most calculations, it is estimated that 23% of the dietary heme iron is absorbed [6]. The absorption of non-heme iron (iron in all other foods) is lower and is affected by the meal composition (other foods present). A person with 500 mg of iron stores would absorb 3 to 8% of the dietary non-heme iron. Non-heme iron makes up 85 to 90% of the iron intake in Western diets [11,12].

In addition to the individual's iron stores, the type of iron consumed, and the accompanying foods, there is limited evidence that training may affect iron absorption. In iron-deficient male distance runners, iron absorption was 16.4% compared to 30% in male controls with depleted iron stores [13]. Thus, concurrent training may reduce iron absorption even if subjects are iron deficient.

How much dietary iron do we need? The typical daily recommendations (RDA = Recommended Dietary Allowance) are 18 mg/day for women and 10 mg/day for men [9]. To meet the iron needs of most women, WHO (World Health Organization) recommends that 2.8 mg of iron should be absorbed daily [14]. These recommended amounts are not always easy to obtain. Normally, iron

Table 14.3. Theoretical Iron Absorption Chart

Caloric Intake (kcal/day)	mg Iron Available (× 6 mg iron/1000 kcal)*	mg Iron Absorbed 10%	20%	30%
1000	6	0.6	1.2	1.8
1582[a]	10	1.0	2.0	3.0
2000	12	1.2	2.4	3.6
2514[b]	15	1.5	3.0	4.5
3000	18	1.8	3.6	5.4
4000	24	2.4	4.8	7.2

a = average caloric intakes for adult women [15, 9]
b = average caloric intakes for adult men [15, 9]
* = from Cook, J. D. [4]

intake is directly proportional to caloric intake. Table 14.3 shows the theoretical caloric intakes required for various amounts of iron being absorbed at different rates. For the average non-exercising woman to meet either the WHO or the RDA recommendations, she would have to take in 2500 kcal (assuming a rather high 20% absorption) or 3000 kcal/day, respectively. To meet their iron needs, many women would have to take in more calories than they expend. Generally, women do tend to absorb a higher percentage of their iron intake than men because of their lower iron stores. Nevertheless, most women have lower iron intakes than what is recommended [9], ranging from about 10-15 mg/day [15,16,17]. The implications of lower iron intakes along with other factors which may affect body iron status are discussed in subsequent sections.

Iron Losses

Because red cells survive in the circulation for approximately 120 days, and there are 4 to 6 million red blood cells, there is considerable red cell turnover, which requires continuous red cell and hemoglobin production. The daily red cell loss is less than 1% of the red cell mass. This represents about 25 mg of iron in hemoglobin turnover. However, when red cells are phagocytized after about 120 days, the iron portions of the molecules are recaptured via the reticuloendothelial system and can be reused. Therefore, it is not necessary to replace all 25 mg of iron from RBC destruction [18].

Normal body iron losses for men are approximately 0.9 mg/day. Besides the normal iron losses, the average adult woman loses an additional 40 to 45 ml of blood per menstrual period which equals about 14 to 15 mg of iron per month. This brings the average iron losses of women to about 1.4 to 1.5 mg/day [8]. However, iron loss from menstrual flow is extremely variable. More importantly, many women have much larger iron losses because of heavy menstrual flow. The average losses in 459 women (19 studies) were 8 to 38 mg of iron per period [19]. The median loss was 0.5 mg/day averaged over the month. However, about 10% of women have iron losses from menstruation above a daily average of 1.4 mg [14] resulting in much larger daily iron losses (over 2.0 mg/day). The larger iron losses of women help explain why they tend to absorb a higher percentage of their iron intake than do men in an attempt to help maintain their iron balance. However, because most women already absorb a higher percentage of their iron intake, they have less reserve capacity for increasing iron absorption to the maximum of about 25% to meet any additional needs [2].

There are other potential sources of iron loss. Every 500 ml blood contains about 250 mg iron. If someone lost or gave 500 ml of blood, he/she would have to absorb an additional 0.7 mg/day for a year to replace that amount of body iron. Sweat is normally considered a negligibly route of iron loss [14,19]. However, profuse sweating may result in a loss of 0.4 to 1.0 mg iron/day [13,20]. Thus, sweat loss during exercise may considerably increase body iron losses [21].

Body Iron Holdings

The total body iron holdings of about 4 gm are divided into several compartments (Table 14.2). (Values may vary depending on the reference used.) Red cell iron (hemoglobin) contains about 65% of the total body iron. Very little iron (0.1%) is in transit in the blood (transport iron). Storage iron holds about 20 to 27% of the body's iron. Iron in other tissues (such as muscle) accounts for an additional 5% of the body's iron in myoglobin (4%) and heme compounds (cytochromes, 1%).

Women have fewer red blood cells, lower hematocrits (packed cell volume = PCV), and lower hemoglobin concentrations than men (Table 14.4). However, the largest sex difference in body iron holdings is in the iron stores (Table 14.2). Men have approximately 1000 mg stored iron compared to 300 to 400 mg for women [4,22]. Cook and Finch [23] determined that 50% of the women in their study had less than 300 mg of stored iron. In other studies, scant or no iron stores have been found in about 10 to 30% of the women

Table 14.4. Normal Blood Values for Iron-Related Compounds

	Men	Women
RBC × 10⁶	5.4 ± 0.7	4.8 ± 0.6
Hgb (g/dl)	16.0 ± 2	14.0 ± 2
Hct (%)	47 ± 5	42 ± 5
MCV (μm^3)	87 ± 7	90 ± 9
SeFe ($\mu g/dl$)	80–160	60–135
TIBC ($\mu g/dl$)	250–350	250–350
% SAT	< 20	< 20
Ferritin (ng/ml)	< 25	< 25
FEP ($\mu g/dlRBCs$)	> 100	> 100

[4,19,24,25]. The lower iron stores in women are evidence that the higher percentage of iron absorption by most women does not fully compensate for their lower iron intake [2] and greater iron losses.

ASSESSMENT OF IRON STATUS

The assessment of iron status is typically described by three areas: (1) red cell iron, (2) transport iron, and (3) storage iron. Red cell iron is reflected by several variables with hemoglobin concentration being the most important. Other variables include RBC number, hemoglobin concentration, hematocrit, and mean cell volume and the related calculations of mean corpuscular hemoglobin and mean corpuscular hemoglobin concentration. Unfortunately, the values for these blood variables are not affected significantly until iron stores are depleted, and therefore, they are not sensitive indicators of impending iron depletion. The average values for red blood cell number and hemoglobin are shown in Table 14.4.

In addition to the iron in red blood cells, the fluid portion of the blood (serum) also contains iron being transported via transferrin, a reusable protein carrier. Iron in serum represents dietary iron absorbed from the intestinal mucosa, iron recouped from RBC and Hb breakdown, and iron being carried to iron requiring tissues. Approximately 30 mg of iron are carried to and from various sites of utilization per day [26].

Transport iron measures consist of the total amount of iron in the serum (serum iron = SeFe), the amount of transferrin available to bind iron for transportation (Total Iron Binding Capacity = TIBC), and the percentage of transferrin that is saturated with iron (percentage of transferrin saturation = % Sat). Both SeFe and TIBC fluctuate diurnally, and SeFe may be affected by the menstrual cycle [19,27]. Consequently, SeFe by itself is not a strong indicator of iron [27,28]. The calculation of transferrin saturation is often a better reflection of iron status than SeFe or TIBC.

The best reflection of body iron status, however, is iron stores. Iron is stored primarily as ferritin (a short-term reservoir) and also as hemosiderin (a long-term" reservoir) [29].

Techniques for the assessment of iron stores are relatively difficult. The traditional measure has been staining of a bone marrow biopsy sample for iron—a highly invasive and only semiquantitative technique. Two other less traumatic methods (blood measurements for serum ferritin and free erythrocyte porphyrin) have been used to indicate iron stores. Serum ferritin is highly correlated to the amount of bone marrow iron but also rises to normal levels after a few days of iron therapy [30]. Free erythrocyte porphyrin (FEP) can also accurately reflect the level of iron stores. The last step in heme synthesis is the combination of iron and protoporphyrin. When iron supply is insufficient, heme synthesis cannot be completed, and unused (free) porphyrin accumulates in the red cell [30,31]. The amount of free erythrocyte porphyrin in the blood increases when iron stores in bone marrow diminish. FEP concentration reflects the adequacy of iron supply because it integrates iron supply and demand [32].

IRON DEFICIENCY

Iron deficiency is the most common nutritional deficiency in the world. Stages of iron deficiency are depicted in Figure 14.3. Iron deficiency is defined as a reduction or disappearance of body iron stores, and it may exist with or without anemia [33]. Anemia is typically defined as a hemoglobin level below 12 g/dl for women and 14 g/dl for men. (Values may vary slightly depending on the reference used.) Iron deficiency anemia does not appear until iron stores are depicted or nearly depleted. Consequently, as mentioned earlier, hemoglobin concentration is not a sensitive indicator of iron deficiency. Hemoglobin levels may be in the "normal" range

	Stores	Marrow Stain	Ferritin μg/l blood	FEP μg/dl RBC's	% SAT	HB g/dl blood
GOOD	600	+2	60	75	35	14
SUBOPTIMAL	200	+1	20	75	35	14
DEFICIENCY						
prelatent	120	0	<12	75	35	14
latent	0	0	<12	100	20	14
deficient erythropoiesis	-150	0	<12	>100	<16	13
ANEMIA						
early	-300	0	<12	>160	<16	<12
late	-600	0	<12	>160	<16	<12

Figure 14.3. Stages of iron deficiency.

although iron stores are very low. Conversely, a low hemoglobin level does not always mean that iron deficiency exists. Some people have values at the low end of the normal range, but those values are actually "normal" for them. Garby et al. [34] found that 30% of their subjects would have been wrongly classified as anemic based on their hemoglobin and hematocrit (PCV) values.

Iron deficiency can be considered as having three stages which are not always distinct: pre-latent, latent, and overt iron deficiency. In pre-latent iron deficiency, there is no clinical evidence, but the individual is less able to meet any increased draw on existing low iron stores brought about by an imbalance between iron absorption and loss. In latent iron deficiency (sideropenia), a biochemical abnormality, clinical abnormality, or both may occur but no anemia exists. However, both SeFe and % Sat fall. In overt iron deficiency, the iron deficiency is severe enough to produce anemia (decreases in hemoglobin concentration and RBCs) [14,35].

Because of their lower iron stores and greater iron losses, women are in a more precarious state of iron balance, and they exhibit a much higher prevalence of iron deficiency and iron deficiency anemia than men. More than five million women (5 to 20%) in the United States have iron deficiency anemia [36,37,38].

EFFECTS OF TRAINING ON IRON STATUS

Numerous factors may impose above normal draws on iron stores. Among the best recognized of these are growth, pregnancy, and lactation. Additionally, it has been suggested that there may be an iron cost associated with strenous physical training [16,17,39, 40,41]. The following section will focus on the effects of training on body iron status by examining the various body iron compartments.

Training and Red Cell Iron

The effects of training on red cell iron variables are important to athletes because oxygen carrying capacity of blood can affect performance in many sport activities. The term "sports anemia" [42] has been used to describe both the blood variable (Hb, Hct, and RBC) decreases associated with training and the low-normal hematological values of some athletes. This term, sports anemia, is a misnomer because the blood variable reductions are relatively small and do not result in clinical anemia. The RBCs tend to be of normal size (normocytic) and contain a normal amount of hemoglobin (normochromic)—conditions different from iron deficiency anemia. Thus, the term "anemia" is not appropriate. Nevertheless, it will be used periodically throughout this chapter because of the frequency of use in the literature.

In the early 1900s, Braun [43] observed that training in dogs resulted in a decrease in the number of RBCs and Hct and Hb level. Generally, evidence regarding the training influence on Hb and RBCs in humans is contradictory. Some studies have shown decreases in Hb and RBCs with training [40,44,45] whereas other studies have found no changes in these variables when pre- and post-training samples were compared [46,47,48]. Other evidence suggests that initial decreases in Hb and RBCs at the beginning of training are transient and that values return to initial levels later in training [16,17,41,42]. Apparently the timing and frequency of measurements are important in being able to observe any blood variable changes with training. According to Yoshimura et al. [49], there is a close correlation between the development of sports anemia and the intensity and duration of physical activity. However, sports anemia has been observed with sustained repetitive work levels of 35% of maximal oxygen consumption [50]. Large and/or sudden increases in physical activity have also resulted in decreases in RBCs and Hb concentrations [17,41,42,49,50,51,52,53,54,55]. Nevertheless, sports anemia did not occur in a group of previously highly trained women runners who increased their mileage only slightly (from about 45 mile/week to about 55 mile/week [56] nor in two groups of male runners (active and recreational runners) who ran four miles at 75% of maximal oxygen consumption every other day [57].

Some studies report that athletes have "suboptimal" Hb and Hct values or values lower than those for less active, normal, and even some training populations [39,58,59,60,61,62,63,64,65,66]. Some evidence suggests that endurance athletes, mainly runners, have a higher incidence of suboptimal hematological values than other athletes [65]. Other studies have compared hematological variables between athletes and nonathletes and found no differences [58,64, 67]. Data from the Sports Physiology Laboratory of the United States Olympic Committee [68] (Figure 14.4) show values well within normal ranges for Hb concentration (and also RBCs and Hct) of athletes in a variety of sports. Some studies have even observed higher than average hemoglobin values in athletes. Women cross-country runners had a mean Hb level of 15 g/dl [69], and the U.S. Nordic Ski team had hemoglobin values of 14.3 and 16 g/dl for women and men, respectively [70]. Such values would be considered just slightly above average for both sexes. Although the data from various studies are not consistent, most red cell values reported for athletes fall well within the normal ranges.

There are several possible explanations for the discrepancies in observations from the literature which include the following: (1) the initial iron status of the subjects (including iron stores and red cell values), i.e., the subjects' susceptibility to iron imbalance; (2) the initial fitness level or state of training of the individuals examined; (3) the type, intensity, and duration of training; (4) the amount of (sudden) increase in training; and (5) diet (especially iron intake) not only prior to but during training.

Several possible explanations may be offered for the decreases in Hb, Hct, and RBCs sometimes observed with training or the low-normal values of some athletes: (1) plasma volume increase, (2) increased RBC destruction, and (3) decreased red cell production. To our knowledge, there is no evidence of a decreased red cell production with physical training although inadequate iron intake/absorption could lead to these circumstances. Larger than normal blood volumes and plasma volumes have been reported for athletes as well as increases in blood volume with training [45,58,71,72,73, 74,75]. Total body hemoglobin increases have also been noted [58,72,75]. Nevertheless, such findings are not consistent and the

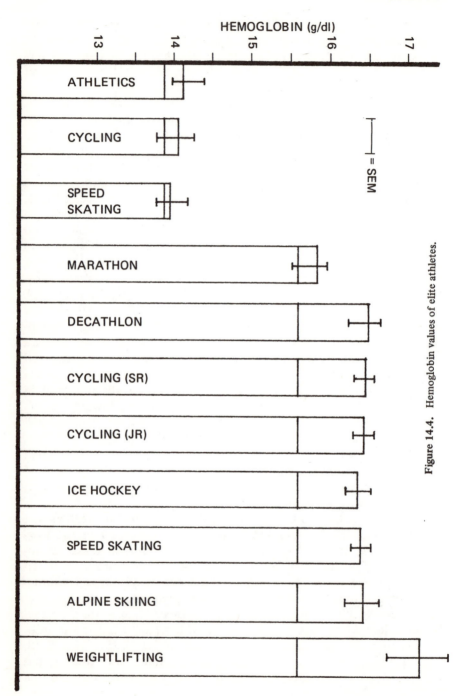

Figure 14.4.   Hemoglobin values of elite athletes.

effects of training on blood volume are not clear [72,75,76,77,78, 79,80]. With an increase in blood (plasma) volume and no change in red cell mass, hemoglobin and other values would appear to be lowered, i.e., a hemodilution effect. However, plasma volume increase can not completely account for the amount of change in many blood variables with training nor the fact that some blood variables increase while others decrease [41].

There is evidence to suggest that reductions in RBC and Hb levels with some types of training occur, at least in part, because of increased red cell destruction. Some supportive evidence for the red cell destruction theory comes from measures of red cell fragility, reticulocytes, and red cell size [17,41,49] although, again, findings are not consistent [50,51,53,56,57]. It has been theorized that an increase in RBC destruction may be due to (1) physical trauma (such as in boxing, marching, running, etc.), (2) wear and tear on red cells because of rapid circulation through capillaries resulting in a weakening of the structural integrity of the red cell membrane, (3) elevated body temperatures associated with exercise, (4) mechanical compression (trauma) of RBCs by muscles during contraction or from body weight in weight bearing activities, and (5) chemical stress, including increased acidosis during exercise or a hemolytic factor, lysolecithin, which is released from the spleen in response to adrenalin secretion [17,41,42,50,52]. An increase in red cell destruction could increase urinary iron excretion [22] and thereby increase iron requirements.

Yoshimura et al. [49] postulated that hemolysis is an adaptation to hard muscular exercise in which hemoglobin freed from destroyed erythrocytes is used for myoglobin accumulation in skeletal muscle. However, if dietary protein was sufficient (1 g/kg body weight/day with 60% animal protein or 2 g/kg/day with 30% animal protein), the incidence of sports anemia was decreased or at least the changes in hematological indices were less and recovery was faster [49]. Data on dietary protein intake in the United States indicates that protein constitutes 10 to 15% of the customary diet [81] and that protein consumption exceeds 1 g/kg/day [15]. Analyses of athletes' diets suggest a higher than average caloric intake and a high percentage of protein. Consequently, protein intakes of athletes often exceed 1.5 g/kg/day (unpublished observations).

The evidence suggests that sports anemia or a diminished oxygen carrying capacity (oxygen per unit of blood) is a possible outcome of strenuous training in some individuals. Nevertheless, a diminished oxygen carrying capacity may not necessarily influence the rate of oxygen delivery, oxygen utilization, or performance. However, if reductions in red cell and hemoglobin levels occur, there may be an increased iron need because red cell production must be higher than usual to reestablish a hematological status that is normal for that individual. Enhanced erythropoietic activity can place a substantial draw on iron stores. As long as stores are adequate and iron absorption is sufficient, it is unlikely that iron depletion would occur. However, for women, who frequently have low iron stores, high iron losses, and low iron intakes, any additional stress including an iron cost with training could be deleterious.

Training and Iron Transport

Measures of iron transport (SeFe, TIBC, and % Sat) have also been investigated in relation to training. Generally, studies indicate that the frequency of low SeFe values is slightly higher in athletes than in the "normal" (nonathletic) population. De Wijn [39] found low SeFe values (70 μg/dl) in 9% of male and 22.5% of female Dutch athletes, and 5% of the men and 15% of the women showed signs of latent iron deficiency. In nine male Finnish biathalonists, four had latent or borderline iron deficiency [64]. Low SeFe values have been noted in women field-hockey players [82] and other training populations [58]. However, Ehn et al. [13] found normal SeFe values in male runners. Significant decreases in SeFe during training [16,40] have been noted in women in some studies whereas other studies have not observed decreases when comparing pre- and post-training values [46,48,83].

Transferrin concentration (TIBC) has been shown to increase during training [16,84,85,86] suggesting a positive influence on iron transport to tissues when exercise stress occurs [84]. However, SeFe or TIBC values are not strong indicators of iron deficiency. The percentage of transferrin saturation, a more sensitive indicator of iron deficiency, has been found to be normal in some studies of athletes and low in others [39,87]. Low percentage of transferrin saturation values were observed in women distance runners [88]. Examination of % Sat values of elite women track and field athletes [67] showed that 2 out of 20 had values below 15% Sat (which is indicative of iron deficiency) and seven out of 20 had % Sat values below 20% (indicative of borderline iron deficiency). None of the three endurance athletes had low iron transport values.

In male and female members of the U.S. Nordic Ski team [70], three out of 10 women had % Sat values below 16%. This is about the same as the 25% observed by Cook et al. [37] in the average female population. None of the men had low transferrin saturation values. (Cook et al. [37] found that 5% of the average male population had low % Sat values.) When a less stringent criteria of 21% Sat was used, 50% of the women skiers and one male skier (10%) had values below (21%). Clement and Asmundson [60] reported that 55% of the women runners and 32% of the male runners in their study had % Sat values below 21%. On the other hand, data from the USOC Sports Physiology Laboratory [68] show that both male and female athletes of the groups examined had transport iron variables within normal ranges (Figure 14.5). (The values for the women speed skaters should be disregarded because of the low number of subjects.)

In a study of highly trained collegiate women runners, there were no changes in % Sat (nor in Hb and RBC values) during their competitive season [56]. However, Frederickson et al. [16] reported decreases of over 20% in SeFe and 25% in % Sat of high-school women cross-country runners during their competitive season. Although the changes were large, they were not statistically significant.

Low % Sat values in athletes indicate an imbalance in iron absorption/loss which could result from inadequate dietary iron or enhanced iron loss associated with training. The implications of low % Sat values for performance in sport are not entirely clear. In reviewing animal data, Dallman [89] suggested that "impaired transport of iron by transferrin can restrict the production of some heme proteins in skeletal muscle to a proportionally similar degree as Hgb (hemoglobin)." An impaired iron transport could, therefore, have an ultimately negative effect on both oxygen carrying capacity of blood (hemoglobin) and oxygen utilization in tissues (myoglobin and cytochromes).

Training and Iron Stores

Do athletes have adequate iron stores? Clement and Asmundsen [60] found that 80% of the women and 29% of the men Canadian distance runners had serum ferritin values below 25 ng/ml. In these runners, iron intake was 18.5 and 12.5 mg/day for the men and women, respectively. Others have noted similarly low ferritin values in women runners where 11 out of 18 had values below 20 ng/ml [90].

In initial observations of the U.S. Nordic Ski team [70], ferritin values were 32 and 51 ng/ml for women and men, respectively, and

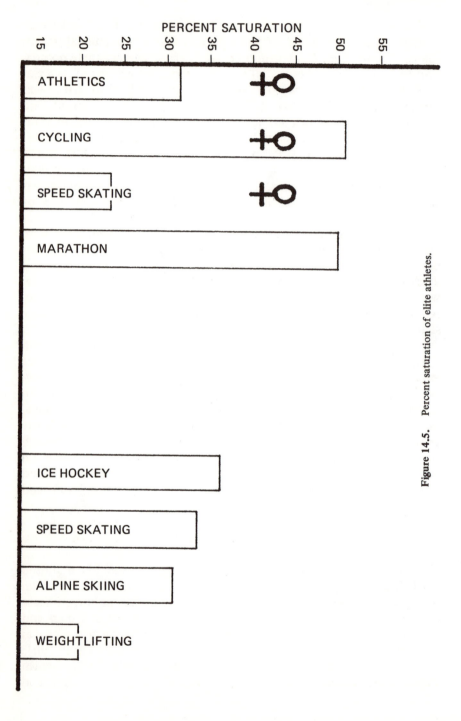

Figure 14.5. Percent saturation of elite athletes.

FEP values were 123 and 116 mg/dl RBCs for the women and men, respectively. The low ferritin values and high FEP values suggest that many of the skiers were using iron at a faster rate than it was being replaced. All 20 skiers had FEP values over 100 μg/dl RBCs whereas in the normal population only 3% of the men and 16% of the women have such values. It appeared that iron depletion was more common in the women skiers than the men skiers but was also a problem for some of the men. Use of iron supplements (18 mg Fe/day) appeared to be beneficial in minimizing iron depletion during the eight-month period, especially among the women skiers. Mean iron intakes were 28.3 and 20.6 mg/day for the men and women, respectively. Decreases in hemoglobin after eight months of training, along with increases in TIBC and FEP values, suggested that the cross-country ski training may reduce the amount of iron available for hemoglobin synthesis. Using the criteria of Cook et al. [37] (three criteria: % Sat less than 16%, FEP values greater than 100 μg/dl RBCs, serum ferritin less than 12 ng/ml), four women skiers out of 10 were classified as iron deficient at sometime during the eight months (and one of these was in the iron supplement group).

A study using FEP levels as an indication of iron stores and iron turnover reported that FEP values increased during the competitive season of high-school women cross-country runners [16]. This data suggested that there was a draw on iron stores associated with training. Other studies have observed low ferritin levels in runners which indicates inadequate iron stores [60,91]. Ferritin values of elite male athletes tested at the USOC Sports Physiology Laboratory (Figure 14.6) were far above borderline values [68]. One of the two groups of women athletes evaluated had mean ferritin values below 25 ng/ml. (There was only one woman speed skater which, therefore, is not a "group.") Approximately 75% (15 out of 20) elite women track and field athletes were iron deficient based on FEP values over 100 μg/dl RBCs [67]. Again, using the criteria of Cook et al. [37], these women would be classified as having marginal iron stores; however, none of the women had FEP values as high as mean values reported for anemic groups.

Bone marrow biopsy information also suggests inadequate iron stores in runners [13,92]. In addition, Ehn et al. [13] found that male runners were using iron approximately twice as fast as the normal adult male. The cause(s) of a faster iron turnover in athletes is (are) not known but may be related to (1) increased RBC destruction and/or (2) increased loss of iron in sweat. Inadequate iron stores may be a consequence of these circumstances.

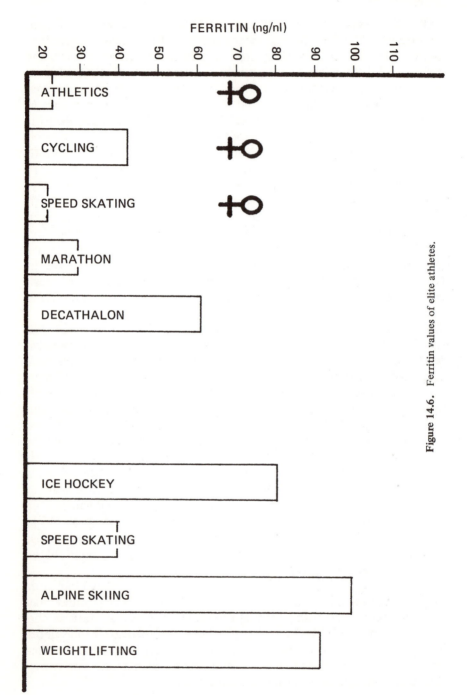

Figure 14.6. Ferritin values of elite athletes.

Implications for Performance

If there is an iron cost associated with some kinds of training, and the individual is in a precarious state of iron balance, an iron deficiency could occur. Iron deficiency may affect oxygen delivery (oxygen carrying capacity) and/or oxygen utilization (cell metabolism) which, in turn, may potentially affect performance in some activities. It is clear that a diminished oxygen carrying capacity negatively affects maximal oxygen consumption, work capacity, and endurance time [93,94,95,96,97,98]. It seems unlikely that the relatively minor decreases in hemoglobin concentration and RBCs sometimes associated with training would have significant effects on performance in most sports. Although there is potential for affecting performance in endurance tasks, there are compensatory mechanisms which operate to help offset decreases in oxygen carrying capacity such as an increase in 2,3-DPG to promote greater oxygen dissociation from hemoglobin at the tissue level. Increased 2,3-DPG levels have been observed in some women runners who also experienced decreases in hemoglobin concentration and red cell number with training [99]. Thus, minor decreases in hemoglobin concentration may not impair performance and, indeed, may be compensated such that performance is not affected.

When plasma volume expansion is the cause of concentration decreases, the total body hemoglobin may actually still be higher than average. Total body hemoglobin content, maximal oxygen consumption, and body size are all highly correlated with one another [100], i.e., a large body is associated with a large maximal oxygen consumption and a large total body hemoglobin. The advantage of a high total body hemoglobin content is not clear. If hemoglobin concentration is reduced, then oxygen carrying capacity (oxygen per unit of blood) is reduced, and heart rate and/or stroke volume must increase to deliver a given quantity of oxygen. It is apparent that when hemoglobin concentration (as a measure of oxygen carrying capacity) is compared to maximal oxygen consumption, there is no relationship—particularly in homogenous groups [100] such as elite athletes in the same sport [68]. Furthermore, there is apparently no correlation between performance and hemoglobin concentration [69,100].

With iron deficiency, it is possible that performance could be affected by factors other than oxygen carrying capacity—specifically, by factors associated with metabolism. Studies on animals show that iron deficiency diminishes the concentration of myoglobin and cytochromes which may affect aerobic metabolism [101]. Even when the oxygen carrying capacity of iron deficient rats was brought to near normal, treadmill endurance was still significantly impaired and lactic acid levels were elevated [102,103]. Iron therapy of borderline deficient subjects resulted in lower maximal lactic acid production (but no increase in maximal oxygen consumption) [104]. Since high lactate production is typically associated with early fatigue, these data indicate that iron deficiency can negatively affect performance through effects at the tissue level even without a reduction in oxygen carrying capacity.

According to Dallman [89], diminished oxygen carrying capacity and iron deficiency have separate effects on physical performance: "The capacity to utilize oxygen for oxidative phosphorylation appears to be particularly critical to the ability to perform sub-maximal exercise for prolonged periods. In contrast, the capacity to deliver oxygen is more closely associated with the peak work load that can be attained in brief intense exercise." Thus, iron deficiency anemia and/or sports anemia (both of which can result in diminished oxygen carrying capacity) would more likely affect maximal oxygen consumption or work capacity in very strenuous exercise whereas iron deficiency (even without anemia) may have implications for endurance through effects on muscle metabolism.

Recommendations

Based on available information, the following recommendations are presented:

1. Periodically (about 3 to 4 times per year) evaluate iron status in order to note changes in the individual. This is more important than comparisons between individuals. Body weight should be monitored simultaneously with blood variables to identify body weight changes associated with fluid alterations which can affect concentrations of blood variables.

2. Examine iron status by measuring variables in more than one iron compartment. Preferably all three compartments (red cell, transport, and storage iron) should be evaluated because there is little correlation between values in different iron compartments (r values for Hb versus % Sat = 0.09, Hb versus ferritin = 0.19, % Sat versus ferritin = 0.03) [68].

3. Start training or change the intensity of training gradually.
4. Follow basic dietary guidelines [81].
5. Do not attempt large weight losses during strenous training because decreased caloric intake also decreases iron intake. This is particularly important for women.
6. Monitor dietary iron intake as well as other dietary factors influencing iron absorption. Some training individuals may have to choose their diets very carefully to meet their iron needs.
7. Moderate iron supplementation may be useful since inadequate iron intake is fairly common. Nevertheless, while deficiencies may negatively affect performance, iron supplementation does not improve performance in iron-replete individuals [46,47,83]. Limited evidence suggests that iron supplementation may help prevent a diminishing of iron status during strenuous training [70].

CONCLUSIONS

Sports anemia is usually a transient condition which occurs with some types and levels of training. The manifestation of sports anemia may be influenced by previous training, type and amount of training, and the iron status of the individual. Probable contributing factors for sports anemia are (1) increased red blood cell destruction, (2) increased loss of iron in sweat, and (3) inadequate iron intake/ absorption. Although increases in plasma volume could contribute to sports anemia, plasma volume changes alone cannot explain all of the blood variable changes observed. Even when decreases in hemoglobin concentration and red blood cells are not observed, available data suggests an iron cost associated with some types of training. Additional draws on iron stores could have health implications for individuals in precarious balance and may require iron supplementation. It is unlikely that sports anemia would significantly affect performance in most sports. However, unmatched long-term iron draws may have more serious implications for health and/or performance. Furthermore, iron deficiency may affect metabolic function. Recommendations to monitor iron-related blood variables, nutritional intake, and training are made in view of a potential iron cost associated with some types of strenuous training, especially running. Because women have lower iron intakes, greater iron losses, and lower iron stores than men, the strenuously training woman may be at greater risk and more prone to any potentially negative effects of training on iron stores.

REFERENCES

1. Dallman, P. R. Tissue effects of iron deficiency. In A. Jacobs and M. Wormood (Eds.), *Iron in biochemistry and medicine* (pp. 437-475). New York: Academic Press, 1974.

2. Munro, H. N. Iron absorption and nutrition. *Fed. Proc., 36,* 2015-2016, 1977.

3. Fairbanks, V. F., Fahey, J. L., and Beutler, E. *Clinical disorders in iron metabolism.* New York: Grune Stratton, 1971.

4. Cook, J. D. Nutritional anemia. Contemporary Nutrition. (General Mills Nutrition Department). *8*(4), 1-2, 1983.

5. Moore, C. V. Iron nutrition. In F. Gross (Ed.), *Iron metabolism* (pp. 241-255). Berlin: Springer-Verlag, 1964.

6. Monsen, E. R., Hallberg, L., Layrisse, M., Hegsted, D. M., Cook, J. D., Mertz, W., and Finch, C. A. Estimation of available dietary iron. *Am. J. Clin. Nutr., 31,* 134-141, 1978.

7. Monsen, E. R., and Balintfy, J. L. Calculating dietary iron bioavailability: Refinement and computerization. *J. Am. Dietetic Assoc., 80,* 307-311, 1982.

8. Verloop, M. C. Iron depletion without anemia: A controversial subject. *Blood, 36,* 657-671, 1970.

9. NAS (National Academy of Sciences). Food and Nutrition Board. *Recommended dietary allowances (9th ed.).* Washington, DC: NAS, 1980.

10. Cook, J. D., and Monsen, E. R. Food iron absorption in human subjects. 111. Comparison of the effect of animal proteins on nonheme iron absorption. *Am. J. Clin. Nutr., 29,* 859-867, 1976.

11. Bull, N. L., and Buss, D. H. Haem and non-haem iron in British household diets. *J. Human Nutr., 34,* 141-145, 1980.

12. Hallberg, L. Bioavailable nutrient density: A new concept applied in the interpretation of food iron absorption data. *Am. J. Clin. Nutr., 34,* 2242-2247, 1981.

13. Ehn, L., Carlmark, B., and Hoglund, S. Iron status in athletes involved in intense physical activity. *Med. Sci. Sports Exer., 12,* 1-64, 1980.

14. Baker, S. J., and DeMaeyer, E. M. Nutritional anemia: Its understanding and control with special reference to the work of the World Health Organization. *Am. J. Clin. Nutr., 32,* 368-417, 1979.

15. Abraham, S., Carroll, M. D., Dresser, C. M., and Johnson, C. L. Dietary intake findings. *Vital Health Stat., 11,* 1-74, 1977.

16. Frederickson, L. A., Puhl, J. L., and Runyan, W. S. Effects of training on indices of iron status of young female cross-country runners. *Med. Sci. Sports Exer., 15,* 271-276, 1983.

17. Puhl, J. L., and Runyan, W. S. Hematological variations during aerobic training of college women. *Res. Q. Exer. Sport, 51,* 533-541, 1980.
18. Guyton, A. C. *Textbook of medical physiology.* Philadelphia: W. B. Saunders Co., 1976.
19. Bowering, J., Sanchez, A. M., and Irwin, M. I. A conspectus of research on iron requirements of man. *J. Nutr., 106,* 985-1074, 1976.
20. Consolazio, C. F., Matoush, L. O., Nelson, R. A., Harding, R. S., and Canham, J. E. Excretion of sodium, potassium, magnesium and iron in human sweat and the relation of each to balance and requirements. *J. Nutr., 79,* 407-415, 1963.
21. Vellar, O. D. Studies on sweat losses of nutrients. I. Iron content of whole body sweat and its association with other sweat constituents, serum iron levels, hematological indices, body surface area and sweat rate. *Scand. J. Clin. Lab. Invest., 21,* 157-167, 1968.
22. Conrad, M. E., and Barton, J. C. Factors affecting iron balance. *Am. J. Hematol., 10,* 199-225, 1981.
23. Cook, J. D., and Finch, C. A. Assessing iron status of a population. *Am. J. Clin. Nutr., 32,* 2115-2119, 1979.
24. Monsen, E. R., Kuhn, I. N., and Finch, C. A. Iron status of menstruating women. *Am. J. Clin. Nutr., 20,* 842-849, 1967.
25. Scott, D. E., and Pritchard, J. A. Iron deficiency in healthy young college women. *J. Am. Med. Assoc., 199,* 147-150, 1967.
26. Huff, R. L., Hennessy, T. G., Austin, R. E., Garcia, J. F., Roberts, B. M., and Lawrence, J. H. Plasma and red cell iron turnover in normal subjects and in patients having various haematopoietic disorders. *J. Clin. Invest., 29,* 1041, 1950.
27. Zilva, J. F., and Patston, V. J. Variations in serum-iron in healthy women. *Lancet, i,* 459-462, 1966.
28. Bainton, D. F., and Finch, C. A. The diagnosis of iron deficiency anemia. *Am. J. Med., 37,* 62-70, 1964.
29. Harrison, P. M. Ferritin and Haemosiderin: Structure and function. In A. Jacobs and M. Worwood (Eds.), *Iron in biochemistry and medicine* (pp. 73-114). New York: Academic Press, 1974.
30. Thomas, W. J., Koenig, H. M., Alton, A. L., and Green, R. Free erythrocyte porphyrin: Hemoglobin ratios, serum ferritin, and transferrin saturation levels during treatment of infants with iron-deficiency anemia. *Blood, 49,* 455-462, 1977.
31. Piomelli, S., Brickman, A., and Carlos, E. Rapid diagnosis of iron deficiency by measurement of free erythrocyte porphyrins and hemoglobin: The FEP/hemoglobin ratio. *Pediatrics, 57,* 136-141, 1976.
32. Langer, E. E., Haining, R. G., Labbe, R. F., Jacobs, P., Crosby, E. F., and Finch, C. A. Erythrocyte protoporphyrin. *Blood, 40,* 112-128, 1972.
33. Mertz, W. Mineral elements: New perspectives. *J. Am. Dietetic Assoc., 77,* 258-263, 1980.
34. Garby, L., Irnell, L., and Werner, I. Iron deficiency in women of fertile age in a Swedish community: Estimation of prevalence based on response to iron supplementation. *Acta Med. Scand., 185,* 113-117, 1969.

35. Cook, J. Clinical evaluation of iron deficiency. *Seminars in Hematology*, *19*, 6-18, 1982.

36. Abraham, S., Lowenstein, F. W., and Johnson, C. L. Preliminary findings of the first health and nutrition examination survey, United States, 1971-1972: Dietary intake and biochemical findings. DHEW Publication No. (HRA) 74-1219-1, 1974.

37. Cook, J. D., Finch, C. A., and Smith, N. J. Evaluation of the iron status of a population. *Blood*, *48*, 449-455, 1976.

38. Fairhurst, E., Dale, T. L. C., and Ridge, B. D. A comparison of anemia and storage iron deficiency in working women. *Proc. Nutr. Soc.*, *36*, 98a, 1977.

39. de Wijn, J. F., De Jongste, J. L., Mosterd, W., and Willebrand, D. Hemoglobin, packed cell volume, serum iron and iron binding capacity of selected athletes during training. *Nutr. Metab.*, *13*, 129-139, 1971.

40. Kilbom, A. Physical training in women. *Scand. J. Clin. Lab. Invest.*, *28* (Suppl. 119), 1-34, 1971.

41. Puhl, J. L., Runyan, W. S., and Kruse, S. J. Erythrocyte changes during training in high school women cross-country runners. *Res. Q. Exer. Sport*, *52*, 484-494, 1981.

42. Yoshimura, H. Anemia during physical training (sports anemia). *Nutr. Rev.*, *28*, 251-253, 1970.

43. Braun, G. O. Blood destruction during exercise. *J. Exp. Med.*, *36*, 481-489, 1922.

44. Brown, B. S., Moore, G. C., Kim, C. K., and Phelps, R. E. Physiological and hematological changes among basketball players during preseason. *Res. Q.*, *45*, 257-262, 1974.

45. Oscai, L. B., Williams, B. T., and Hertig, B. A. Effect of exercise on blood volume. *J. Appl. Physiol.*, *24*, 622-624, 1968.

46. Cooter, G. R., and Mowbray, K. W. Effects of iron supplementation and activity on serum iron depletion and hemoglobin levels in female athletes. *Res. Q.*, *49*, 114-118, 1978.

47. Weswig, P. H., and Winkler, W., Jr. Iron supplementation and hematological data of competitive swimmers. *J. Sports Med. Physical Fitness*, *14*, 112-119, 1974.

48. Wirth, J. C., Lohman, T. G., Avallone, J. P., Jr., Shire, T., and Boileau, R. A. The effect of physical training on the serum iron levels of college-age women. *Med. Sci. Sports*, *10*, 223-226, 1978.

49. Yoshimura, H., Inoue, T., Yamada, T., and Shiraki, K. Anemia during hard physical training (sports anemia) and its causal mechanism with special reference to protein nutrition. *World Rev. Nutr. Diet*, *35*, 1-86, 1980.

50. Radomski, M. W., Sabiston, B. H., and Isoard, P. Development of "sports anemia" in physically fit men after daily sustained submaximal exercise. *Aviat. Space Environ. Med.*, *51*, 41-45, 1980.

51. Dressendorfer, R. H., Wade, C. E., and Amsterdam, E. A. Development of pseudoanemia in marathon runners during a 20-day road race. *J. Am. Med. Assoc.*, *246*, 1215-1218, 1981.

52. Lindemann, R., Ekanger, R., Opstad, P. K., Nummestad, M., and Ljosland, R. Hematological changes in normal men during prolonged severe exercise. *Am. Corr. Ther. J.*, *32*, 107-111, 1978.

53. Rasch, P. J., Hamby, J. W., and Burns, H. J., Jr. Protein dietary supplementation and physical performance. *Med. Sci Sports*, *1*, 195-199, 1969.

54. Shiraki, K., Yoshimura, H., and Yamada, T. Anemia during physical training and physical performance. Proceedings of the XXth World Congress in Sports Medicine, Melbourne, 1974.

55. Sumiyoshi, K. A. A study on the changes of body fluid and the circulatory system of athletes. In K. Kato (Ed.), *Proceedings of the International Congress of Sport Sciences* (pp. 362-363). Tokyo: The Japanese Union of Sport Sciences, 1964.

56. Puhl, J. L., and Runyan, W. S. Hematology of women cross-country runners during training. *Med. Sci. Sports Exer.*, *12*, 108, 1980.

57. Hanson, P. G., Buhr, B., Sarnwick, R., and Shahidi, N. A. Exercise hemolysis in trained and untrained runners. *Med. Sci. Sports*, *10*, 48, 1978.

58. Brotherhood, J., Brozovic, B., and Pugh, L. G. C. Haematological status of middle- and long-distance runners. *Clin. Sci. Molec. Med.*, *48*, 139-145, 1975.

59. Clement, D. B., Asmundson, and Medhurst, C. W. Hemoglobin values: Comparative survey of the 1976 Canadian Olympic team. *Can. Med. Assoc. J.*, *117*, 614-616, 1977.

60. Clement, D. B., and Asmundson, R. C. Nutritional intake and hematological parameters in endurance runners. *Phys. Sportsmed*, *10*, 37-43, 1982.

61. Clement, D. B., Taunton, J. E., and Poskitt, K. Iron deficiency anemia in a distance runner. *Can. Family Physician*, *28*, 1008-1010, 1982.

62. Hiramatsu, S. Studies on the cause of erythrocyte destruction in muscular exercise (changes in erythrocyte properties in sports training and their physiological significance). Report 1. *Acta Haematol. Jap.*, *23*, 843-851, 1960.

63. Hunding, A., Jordal, R., and Paulev, P. E. Runners anemia and iron deficiency. *Acta Med. Scand.*, *209*, 315-318, 1981.

64. Sarviharju, P. J., Rahkila, P., Vihko, V., Rajala, M., and Karvinen, E. Iron deficiency of selected top-level biathalonists during training. *IRCS Med. Sci.*, *3*, 295, 1975.

65. Stewart, G. A., Steel, J. E., and Toyne, A. H. Observations of the haematology and the iron and protein intake of Australian Olympic athletes. *Med. J. Austr.*, *2*, 1339-1343, 1972.

66. Willan, P. L. T., Bagnall, K. M., Mahon, M., and Kellett, D. W. Some haematological characteristics of competitive swimmers. *Brit. J. Sports Med.*, *15*, 238-241, 1981.

67. Puhl, J. L., Hagerman, G. R., Brown, C. H., and Van Handel, P. J. Hematological and iron status of elite track and field women. *Med. Sci. Sports Exer.*, *14*, 154, 1982.

68. Puhl, J. L., Van Handel, P. J., Williams, L., Bradley, P. W., and Harms, S. J. Iron status of elite athletes. United States Olympic Committee, Sports Physiology Report (unpublished).
69. Runyan, W. S., and Puhl, J. L. Relationships between selected blood indices and competitive performance in college women cross-country runners. *J. Sports Med. Physical Fitness*, *20*:207-212, 1980.
70. Haymes, E. M., Puhl, J. L., and Temples, T. E. Training for cross-country skiing and iron status. Paper presented at ACSM. Montreal, Canada, 1983.
71. Akgun, N., Tartaroglu, N., Durosoy, F., and Kocaturk, E. The relationship between the changes in physical fitness and in total blood volume in subjects having regular and measured training. *J. Sports Med. Physical Fitness*, *14*, 73-77, 1974.
72. Dill, D. B., Braithwaite, K., Adams, W. C., and Bernauer, E. M. Blood volume of middle-distance runners: Effect of 2,300-m altitude and comparison with non-athletes. *Med. Sci. Sports*, *6*, 1-7, 1974.
73. Fortney, S. M., and Senay, L. C., Jr. Effect of training and heat acclimation on exercise responses of sedentary females. *J. Appl. Physiol: Respirat. Environ. Exer. Physiol.*, *47*, 978-984, 1979.
74. Holmgren, A., Mossfeldt, F., Sjöstrand, T., and Ström, G. Effect of training on work capacity, total hemoglobin, blood volume, heart volume and pulse rate in recumbent and upright positions. *Acta Physiol. Scand.*, *50*, 72-83, 1960.
75. Kjellberg, S. R., Rudhe, U., and Sjöstrand, T. Increase of the amount of hemoglobin and blood volume in connection with physical training. *Acta Physiol. Scand.*, *19*, 146-151, 1949.
76. Bass, D. E., Buskirk, E. R., and Iampietro, P. F. Comparison of blood volume during physical conditioning, heat acclimatization and sedentary living. *J. Appl. Physiol.*, *12*, 186-188, 1958.
77. Cook, D. R., Gualtier, W. S., Galla, S. J. Body fluid volumes of college athletes and nonathletes. *Med. Sci. Sports*, *1*, 217-220, 1970.
78. Dill, D. B., Hall, F. G., Hall, K. D., Dawson, C., and Newton, J. L. Blood, plasma, and red cell volumes: Age, exercise, and environment. *J. Appl. Physiol.*, *21*, 597-602, 1966.
79. Moore, R., and Buskirk, E. R. Exercise and body fluids. In (W. Johnson (Ed.), *Science and medicine of exercise and sports* (pp. 207-235). New York: Harper and Row, 1960.
80. Scheur, J., and Tipton, C. M. Cardiovascular adaptation to physical training. *Annual Rev. Physiol.*, *39*, 221-251, 1977.
81. ADA (American Dietetic Association). Nutrition and physical fitness. *J. Am. Dietetic Assoc.*, *76*, 437-443, 1980.
82. Haymes, E. M., Harris, D. V., Beldon, M. D., Loomis, J. L., and Nicholas, W. C. The effect of physical activity level on selected hematological variables in adult women. Paper presented at the Research Section of AAHPER, Houston, Texas, 1972.
83. Pate, R. R., Maguire, M., and Van Wyk, J. Dietary iron supplementation in women athletes. *Physic. and Sports Med.*, *7*(9), 81-86, 1979.

84. Haralambie, G. Serum glycoproteins and physical exercise. *Clin. Chim. Acta,* 27, 475–479, 1969.
85. Haralambie, G. Changes of serum glycoprotein levels after long-lasting physical exercise. *Clin. Chim. Acta,* 27, 475–479, 1970.
86. Haralambie, G., and Keul, J. Serum glycoprotein levels in athletes in training. *Experientia,* 26, 959–960, 1970.
87. Haymes, E. M. Iron-deficiency and the active woman. *DGWS Research Reports: Women in Sports,* 2, 91–95, 1973.
88. Plowman, S. A., and McSwegin, P. J. The effects of iron supplementation on female cross country runners. *J. Sports Med.,* 21, 407–416, 1981.
89. Dallman, P. R. Manifestations of iron deficiency. *Seminars in Hematology,* 19, 19–30, 1982.
90. Nickerson, H. J., and Tripp, A. D. Iron deficiency in adolescent cross-country runners. *Physic. and Sports Med.,* 11(6), 60–66, 1983.
91. Dufaux, B., Hoederath, A., Streitberger, Hollman, W., and Assman, G. Serum ferritin, transferrin, haptoglobin and iron in middle- and long-distance runners, elite rowers and professional racing cyclists. *Int. J. Sports Med.,* 2, 43–46, 1981.
92. Wishnitzer, R., Vorst, E., and Berrebi, A. Bone marrow iron depression in competitive distance runners. *Int. J. Sports Med.,* 4, 27–30, 1983.
93. Anderson, H. T., and Barkve, H. Iron deficiency and muscular work performance: An evaluation of the cardio-respiratory function of iron deficient subjects with and without anemia. *Scand. J. Clin. Lab. Invest.,* 25(Suppl. 114), 1–62, 1970.
94. Edgerton, V. R., Bryant, S. L., Gillespie, C. A., and Gardner, G. W. Iron deficiency anemia and physical performance and activity of rats. *J. Nutr.,* 102, 381–400, 1972.
95. Edgerton, V. R., Gardner, G. W., Ohira, Y., Gunawardena, K. A., and Senewiratne, B. Iron-deficiency anemia and its effect on worker productivity and activity patterns. *Br. Med. J.,* 2, 1546–1549, 1979.
96. Ekblom, B., Goldbarg, A. N., and Gullbring, B. Response to exercise after blood loss and reinfusion. *J. Appl. Physiol.,* 33, 175–180, 1972.
97. Gardner, G., Edgerton, V., Senewiratne, B., Barnard, R., and Ohira, Y. Physical work capacity and metabolic stress in subjects with iron deficiency anemia. *Am. J. Clin. Nutr.,* 30, 910–917, 1977.
98. Viteri, F., and Torun, B. Anemia and physical work capacity. *Clinics in Haematology,* 3, 609–626, 1974.
99. Smalley, K. A., Runyan, W. S., and Puhl, J. L. Effect of training on erythrocyte 2,3-diphosphoglycerate in two groups of women cross-country runners. *J. Sports Med. and Phys. Fitness,* 21, 352–358, 1981.
100. Hermansen, L. Oxygen transport during exercise in human subjects: Relative and total hemoglobin content of the blood and maximal oxygen uptake. *Acta Physiol. Scand.,* 90(Suppl.), 37–46, 1974.
101. Siimes, M. A., Refino, C., and Dallman, P. R. Manifestations of iron deficiency at various levels of iron intake. *Am. J. Clin. Nutr.,* 33, 570–574, 1980.

102. Finch, C. A., Miller, L. R., Inamdar, A. R., Person, R., Seiler, K., and Mackler, B. Iron deficiency in the rat. Physiological and biochemical studies of muscle dysfunction. *J. Clin. Invest.*, *58*, 447–453, 1976.

103. Finch, C. A., Gollnick, P. D., Hlastala, M. P., Miller, L. R., Dillman, E., and Mackler, B. Lactic acidosis as a result of iron deficiency. *J. Clin. Invest.*, *64*, 129–137, 1979.

104. Schoene, R. B., Escourrou, P., Robertson, H. T., Nilson, K. L., Parsons, J. R., and Smith, N. J. Iron repletion decreases maximal exercise lactate concentrations in female athletes with minimal iron-deficiency anemia. *J. Lab. Clin. Med.*, *102*, 306–331, 1983.

V.
Nutrition

CHAPTER **15**

Profile of Nutritional Beliefs and Practices of the Elite Athlete

Ann C. Grandjean

"There is no area of nutrition where faddism, misconceptions and ignorance are more obvious than in athletes" [1]. Surveys have indicated that the nutrition knowledge, recommendations, and practices of athletes and members of their support staff are less than optimal [2-7]. However, there is a paucity of data on the nutrition knowledge and/or nutritional practices of elite athletes.

Researchers agree that factual nutrition information should be provided to athletes and their support staff, and coaches and athletes are unquestionably interested in the subject [2,6,7]. But with all the many topics to be covered, where does the sports nutrition educator begin? One of the basic principles of education is to "start where the learner is."

A survey of college athletes was conducted to help identify the discrepancies between what is known and practiced by athletes and what is recommended [8]. Results indicated that athletes felt performance is improved by a high-protein diet and that large amounts of protein are needed to increase muscle mass. The majority of the athletes also felt natural vitamins are superior to synthetic vitamins and that athletes require larger amounts of vitamins than nonathletes. Although most of the athletes surveyed knew the value of water in preventing heat illness and maintaining optimal performance, the majority did not know that an athlete needs to drink more than thirst demands. Survey results also indicated that more information is needed by athletes regarding the use of salt tablets, as 49% of those surveyed thought salt tablets should be taken in hot weather.

DIETARY PROFILES

To help determine actual dietary practices, comprehensive dietary data have been collected on close to 150 athletes. These athletes range in age from 11 to 35 years, in height from 4'8" to 6'5", and in weight from 73 to 310 pounds. They include athletes participating in U.S. Olympic Committee-sponsored programs, football players at the University of Nebraska, a junior gymnastic team competing at the national level, and a professional baseball team.

CALORIC INTAKES

Books and articles on nutrition and athletes often contain such statements as

The biggest difference in nutrition requirements between the athlete and the nonathlete concerns energy, especially during training or conditioning [9].

Table 15.1 Caloric Intakes of Male Athletes by Sport

Sport	Mean	Range
Baseball	4,605	2,086–6,407
Swimming	4,521	3,655–5,233
Football	3,873	1,785–5,787
Judo	3,461	2,497–5,302
Weight Lifting	3,417	1,886–6,085
Hockey	3,082	1,888–4,905
Figure Skating	3,066	2,958–3,174
Diving	2,594	1,987–3,089
Wrestling	1,956	900–3,509

Table 15.2 Calorie Intakes of Female Athletes by Sport

Sport	Mean	Range
Figure Skating	1,800	1,412–2,187
Judo	1,796	1,050–2,406
Gymnastics (juniors)	1,671	1,175–1,924

The unique nutritional requirements of the athlete is his high requirement of energy [10].

Such statements imply that an athlete automatically, because he/she is an athlete, has a high caloric requirement. Our data indicate this is not always the case. The energy requirement of an athlete depends on age, gender, height, weight, body composition, type of sport, physical conditioning, clothing worn, playing surface, environment in which the athletic activity takes place, and the frequency, intensity, and duration of the event or training session [11,12,13]. The daily caloric intakes (individual averages) of the athletes studied to date range from 900 calories to 6,407 calories. The caloric intakes by sport and sex are given in Tables 15.1 and 15.2.

CALORIC DISTRIBUTION

Caloric distribution is one of the dietary concerns of athletes. Various recommendations for determining standards can be used. The dietary goals may be considered for health reasons [14]. Regimens designed to increase glycogen storage may be the standard for endurance athletes [15]. Or for athletes who are increasing

Table 15.3 Caloric Distribution by Sport
(group means)

Sport	% of Calories from			
	CHO	F	P	ALC
Wrestling	53	33	14	neg
Football	43	41	15	1
Weight Lifting	50	31	17	2
Hockey	44	36	19	1
Baseball	40	35	17	8

Table 15.4 Group and Individual Ranges of Caloric Distribution

	% of Calories from			
	CHO	F	P	ALC
Group	40–53	31–41	14–19	neg– 8
Individual	23–69	16–56	9–28	0–28

muscle mass, protein and calorie requirements may be the major concern [16]. Caloric distributions for some of the athletes studied are shown in Table 15.3. The percentage of calories from carbohydrate for some athletes is below that recommended by many nutritionists and sports physiologists. The ranges are even more dramatic if one looks at the caloric distribution of individuals (Table 15.4).

PROTEIN

Many athletes are particularly concerned with the protein content of the diet. Of the athletes studied to date, swimmers have the highest protein consumption at 2.1 grams of protein per kilogram of body weight, and wrestlers the lowest at 1.0 gram per kilogram (Table 15.5). As with caloric distribution, there is great individual variation within each sport (Table 15.6). In reviewing the dietary

Table 15.5 Protein of Athletes in Various Sports

Sport	Grams of Protein/kg
Swimming	2.1
Baseball	1.9
Weight Lifting	1.8
Football	1.8
Diving	1.8
Judo (male)	1.8
Hockey	1.6
Figure Skating (female)	1.5
Gymnastics (junior female)	1.5
Figure Skating (male)	1.4
Judo (female)	1.1
Wrestling	1.0

Table 15.6 Group Means and Ranges of Grams of Protein
Ingested per Kilogram of Body Weight

Sport	Mean	Range
Baseball	1.9	.59–3.66
Weight Lifting	1.8	.77–3.02
Football	1.8	.69–2.8
Wrestling	1.0	.44–2.21

intake data, patterns emerge when the data are analyzed by sport. However, there are great individual differences within each sport.

VITAMINS AND MINERALS

Another standard by which dietary adequacy is often evaluated is the amounts of vitamins and minerals provided, the most commonly used standard being the recommended dietary allowances [13]. Of the athletes studied to date, a wide range of intakes for several nutrients has been found (Table 15.7). The majority of athletes with dietary intakes less than 70% the RDA for more than one nutrient participated in gymnastics or wrestling and did not use dietary supplements.

In the group of junior gymnasts, all had iron intakes of less than 70% the RDA, and 83% had intakes of calcium less than 70% the RDA (Table 15.8). The nutrient most frequently low in the diets of the wrestlers was vitamin A, with 45% of the wrestlers consuming less than 70% the RDA of Vitamin A (Table 15.9). On the other

Table 15.7 Extremes in Intakes of Selected
Nutrients

Nutrient	% RDA
Calcium	14-706
Iron	36-7,494
Vitamin A	27-1,534
Thiamine	33-14,421
Riboflavin	59-12,662
Niacin	26-5,676
Vitamin C	61-8,233

**Table 15.8 Percent of Junior Gymnasts
Consuming Less that 70% RDA for
Selected Nutrients**

Nutrient	Percent Consuming <70% RDA
Iron	100
Calcium	83
Vitamin A	33
Niacin	33
Thiamine	2

hand, some athletes had extremely high intakes of some nutrients (Table 15.7), which for the most part was due to the use of dietary supplements.

DIETARY SUPPLEMENTS

The number of athletes reporting routine use of dietary supplements (52%) was not surprising, However, the high level at which some of the athletes were supplementing was not anticipated. Again, patterns emerge when the data are analyzed by sport (Table 15.10). For the most part, those athletes who use supplements have adequate diets and those with less than adequate diets do not use supplements [17].

The types of supplements used by athletes are presented in Table 15.11. Eight-two percent of the athletes who reported taking

**Table 15.9 Percent Wrestlers Consuming Less
than 70% RDA for Selected Nutrients**

Nutrient	Percent Consuming <70% RDA
Vitamin A	45
Calcium	36
Iron	36
Niacin	36
Thiamine	27
Riboflavin	18
Vitamin C	9

Table 15.10 Percent of Athletes Reporting
Routine Use of Supplements (by Sport)

Sport	Percent
Swimming	80
Baseball	75
Judo (female)	75
Weight Lifting	72
Judo (male)	64
Figure Skating (female)	50
Figure Skating (male)	50
Hockey	38
Wrestling	38
Football	18
Diving	2
Gymnastics (junior female)	0

supplements used vitamin-mineral combinations. Other supplements used, in decreasing order, were vitamin preparations, minerals, protein (powder or tablets), yeast, multinutrient powders or liquids (usually containing carbohydrate, vitamins, and minerals), alfalfa, bee pollen, caffeine (pills), ginseng, lecithin, and wheat germ.

When counseling an athlete who uses supplements, consideration should be given to nutrient deficiencies, toxic levels, and unnecessary supplementation. For athletes consuming less than 70% the RDA of a given nutrient, diet modification is indicated and supplementation

Table 15.11 Types of Supplements Reported
Taken by Athletes

Supplement	Percent
Vitamin/mineral	82
Vitamin	46
Mineral	25
Protein	10
Yeast	6
Multinutrient powder or liquid	3
Alfalfa	1
Bee pollen	1
Caffeine (pills)	1
Ginseng	1
Lecithin	1
Wheat germ	1

should be considered. For athletes consuming extremely high levels of nutrients, toxicity should be a concern [18].

There has been an increase in the number of nonnutritive supplements being used by athletes [17]. Nonnutritive supplements are substances with no demonstrated nutritional value although the substance may be found in naturally occurring foods. Bioflavinoids and pangamic acid (vitamin B_{15}) are two of the nonnutritive supplements commonly promoted for and used by athletes. The use of so-called vitamin B_{15} is propagated by enthusiastic promotions by purveyors and testimonials from public figures, including well-known athletes [19]. One of the disturbing factors about this substance is that there is no such chemical entity as pangamate, pangamic acid, or vitamin B_{15}, and there is no control over compounds sold under these names. The fact that potentially toxic substances are sometimes marketed under these names is dangerous, especially to the athlete who may be tempted to take large amounts [20]. Bioflavinoids ("vitamin P") are another example of nonnutritive supplements [21]. Hesperidin, rutin, and citrin (citrus bioflavinoids) are bioflavinoids frequently found in supplements promoted for athletes. Silica, more commonly known as sand, is even being marketed as a nutritional supplement. It appears that for every element, there is an enthusiastic "pusher," as well as a willing buyer.

REFERENCES

1. Durnin, J. The influence of nutrition. *Can. Med. Assoc. J.*, *96*, 715, 1967.
2. Werblos, J. A., Fox, H. M., and Henneman, A. Nutritional knowledge, attitudes, and food patterns of women athletes. *J. Amer. Diet. Assoc.*, *73*, 242, 1978.
3. Costill, D. L., Sharp, R. L., and Sherman, W. M. A survey of the nutritional habits among collegiate athletes. Project Report from the Human Performance Laboratory, Ball State University, 1982.
4. Cho, M., and Fryer, B. A. Nutritional knowledge of collegiate physical education majors. *J. Amer. Diet. Assoc.*, *65*, 30, 1974.
5. Cho, M., and Fryer, B. A. What foods do physical education majors and basic nutrition students recommended for athletes? *J. Amer. Diet. Assoc.*, *65*, 541, 1974.
6. Wolf, E. M. B., Wirth, J. C., and Lohman, T. G. Nutritional practices of coaches in the big ten. *The Physician and Sports Medicine*, 7, 113, 1979.
7. Bentwegna, A., Kelley, E. J., and Kalenak, A. Diet, fitness, and athletic performance. *The Physician and Sports Medicine*, 7, 99, 1979.

8. Grandjean, A. C., Hursh, L. M., Majure, W. C., and Hanley, D. F. Nutrition knowledge and practices of college athletes. *Medicine and Science in Sports and Exercise, 13*(2), 82, 1981.

9. Darden, E. *The Nautilus Nutrition Book*. Chicago: Contemporary Books, Inc., 1981.

10. Smith, N. J. *Food for Sport*. Palo Alto, CA: Bull Publishing Co., 1976.

11. Horstman, D. H. Nutrition. In W. P. Morgan (Ed.), *Ergogenic Aids and Muscular Performance*. New York: Academic Press, 1972.

12. Konishi, F. *Exercise Equivalents of Foods: A Practical Guide for the Overweight*. Carbondale, IL: Southern Illinois University Press, 1974.

13. National Research Council. *Recommended Dietary Allowances*, (9th ed.). Washington, D.C.: National Academy of Sciences, 1980.

14. Select Committee on Nutrition and Human Needs, United States Senate. *Dietary Goals for the United States*, (2nd ed.). Washington, D.C.: U.S. Government Printing Office, 1977.

15. Costill, D. L., Sherman, W. M., Fink, W. J., Maresh, C., Witten, M., and Miller, J. M. The role of dietary carbohydrates in muscle glycogen resynthesis after strenuous running, *The Amer. J. of Clinical Nutr. 34*, 1831, 1981.

16. Laritcheva, K. A., Yalovaya, N. I., Shubin, V. I., and Smirnov, P. V. Study of energy expenditure and protein needs of top weight lifters. In J. Parizkova and V. A. Rogozkin (Eds.), *Nutrition, Physical Fitness, and Health*. Baltimore, MD: University Park Press, 1978.

17. Grandjean, A. C., and Lolkus, L. Dietary profiles of athletes, Unpublished data, 1983.

18. Miller, D. R., and Hayes K. C. Vitamin excess and toxicity. In J. H. Hathcook (Ed.), *Nutritional Toxicity*. New York: Academic Press, 1982.

19. Food and Drug Administration. Dubunking pangamic acid. F.D.A. Consumer, September, 1978.

20. Smith, N. J. Nutrition and the athlete. *Am. J. Sports. Med., 10*, 253, 1982.

21. Marshall, C. W. *Vitamins and Minerals: Help or Harm?* Philadelphia: George F. Stickley Co., 1983.

CHAPTER **16**

Nutrition and Performance: Carbohydrates, Fluids, and Pregame Meals

Richard B. Parr

Diets and dietary manipulation have shown to compliment training regimens to enhance performance. In their proper perspective, carbohydrate loading, fluid intake, and pregame meals can
contribute significantly to performance. However, diets cannot
replace inadequate training and physical conditioning. Conversely,
poor nutritional practices will jeopardize the highly trained and
skilled athlete's performance. The best insurance policy for nutritional status is a good diet including a variety of foods chosen from
recommended food groups such as the Basic Four (Daily Food
Guide) or the Dietary Exchange List. Under normal dietary conditions it is difficult to create deficiency in any nutrient. Additionally,
vitamin and mineral supplementation has not proven to be beneficial
to athletic performance.

There are, however, three dietary practices that will benefit
performance when practiced in conjunction with events appropriate
to their mechanism of action. The decline in performance when
muscle glycogen stores become depleted has been documented [1–4],
and dietary intervention prior to performance has shown to increase

The Elite Athlete, edited by N. K. Butts, T. T. Gushiken, and B. Zarins. Copyright © 1985
by Spectrum Publications, Inc.

the time to exhaustion. Additionally, decreased body fluids have shown to significantly decrease performance [5-8] while fluid intake prior to and during performance partially counteracts the detrimental effects of dehydration. Finally, inappropriate precompetition meals can interfere with performance.

CARBOHYDRATE UTILIZATION AND LOADING

Substrate utilization for energy during work has been studied over the past 50 years in an attempt to determine the roles of diet in performance. Original studies relied on respiratory exchange to estimate the role of energy substrates for work. Although adjustments were made for lactic acid and buffering mechanisms, the contributions of fat and glycogen for energy were not directly measured. A more accurate yet complicated method employed the measurement of arterio-venous differences in energy substrates and metabolites during exercise [9]. In the 1960s Bergstrom and Hultman [10] developed the needle biopsy technique to study intramuscular glycogen utilization during exercise and subsequent replacement related to a variety of dietary practices. Accumulated research has given the practitioner the background information necessary to confidently develop dietary and training programs for optimal performance. The following discussion will show that (1) exercise does reduce muscle glycogen stores, (2) initial glycogen stores are important to the time of exhaustion, and (3) diet does substantially effect muscle glycogen stores.

The ratio of carbohydrate to fat utilization during work is related to intensity and duration as well as diet, fitness levels, and recruitment of muscle fibers. It is well established that the rate of glycogen utilization increases proportionate to intensity of work [3] (Table 16.1). The shift of carbohydrate utilization at higher intensities is an advantage because of the reduced availability of oxygen at these workloads. At lower workloads where oxygen supply is adequate, fats are more efficiently utilized as the primary energy source. Fat utilization "spares" glycogen for its most efficient use, when oxygen supply is less available. Training then must be specific to the energy substrate required for work and the muscle fibers primarily recruited. Exercise of moderate intensity depletes slow twitch fibers first, followed by fast twitch fibers which would be recruited upon depletion of slow twitch fibers. Fast twitch fibers, on the other hand, are depleted first during high intensity work [11].

Table 16.1. Energy Substrate for Work

Intensity (% $\dot{V}O_2$ max)	Duration	Fiber Type	% Calories CHO	% Calories Fat
200	10 sec.	FT	100	0
120	4 min.	FT		
100	5	FT	90	10
90	30	ST		
80	2 hrs.	ST	80	20
70	4	ST	70	30
60		ST	60	40
50		ST	50	50
40		ST	40	60
30		ST	30	70

The use of carbohydrates for fuel depends largely on diet. Havel et al. [12] showed that when carbohydrates were available, they were the preferred source of energy. They found that fasting subjects used ten percent of the energy required for work from carbohydrates and 50 percent from fats. Their "fed" subjects derived 80 percent of their energy from carbohydrates and 10 percent from fats.

Exercise Reduces Muscle Glycogen Stores

The effects of exercise on muscle glycogen stores have been the focus of much study [2,3,10,11,13] and are summaried in Table 16.2. It is well demonstrated that glycogen stores were reduced proportionately to the intensity and duration of work. When exercise was prolonged until exhaustion at intensities of 70 to 80 percent $\dot{V}O_2$ max, the muscle glycogen stores were nearly depleted [2,3]. The first of these studies were done in Europe using bicycle ergometers. More recently studies in the United States have used running as the mode of exercise and have found similar trends in glycogen depletion but have introduced two important variables: (1) supramaximal intensities and (2) involvement of greater muscle mass. Gollnick et al. [11] used intensities of 150 percent $\dot{V}O_2$ max on an interval basis and found that fast twitch muscle fibers were depleted first followed by slow twitch fibers. It is apparent from this study that intensity of work produces specific metabolic responses, a consideration when developing training programs. Costill et al. [13] found decreases in glycogen content of the vastus lateralis muscle

Table 16.2.   Studies Related to Muscle Glycogen Reduction through Exercise

Study	Mode	Treatment	Results
Hultman, 1966	Bicycle	30 min. light work (300 kpm)	Decrease glycogen stores by 29%
Hermansen, Hultman, and Saltin, 1967	Bicycle	Continuous versus intermittant work	Muscles glycogen depletion: 25% $\dot{V}O_2$max (1 hr) = -.31 g/100 g wet wt.; 54% $\dot{V}O_2$max (1 hr) = -.83 g/100 g wet wt.; 78% $\dot{V}O_2$max (1 hr) = 1.83 g/100 g wet wt.
Bergstrom and Hultman, 1966	Bicycle	One-legged exercise to exhaustion (serial biopsy)	Exercised leg = glycogen depletion of 1.3–1.6 g/100 g wet wt.; nonexercised leg = normal levels of glycogen
Gollnick et al., 1973	Sprint runs	150% $\dot{V}O_2$max 6–1 min. sprints (10 min. rests)	Initial glycogen = 132 mM/kg. Following 1st workout = 106 mM/kg. Following 6th workout = 49 mM/kg. (1st fibers depleted = FT, low oxidative/high glycolytic)
Costill et al., 1971	16.1 km (10 mile) run	80% $\dot{V}O_2$max	Glycogen depletion: soleus = from 2.66 to 1.06 g/100 g wet wt. gastrocnemius = from 2.02 to .66 g/100 g wet wt. vastus lateralis = from 1.87 to .74 g/100 g wet wt.

when running 16 km at 80 percent $\dot{V}O_2$ max, but the decrease was less than that found by other investigators using bicycles as the mode of work [3,10]. Costill et al. [13] further found that the soleus and gastrocnemius muscles reduced their glycogen content to a greater extent than the vastus lateralis. As more muscle groups are involved in exercise, they accept some of the burden of energy supply otherwise given to isolated muscles.

Initial Glycogen Stores Related to Exhaustion

Exhaustion is often associated with significant reduction of muscle glycogen. Initial glycogen stores are important in increasing the time to exhaustion when running at specific intensities. Also, the time to run a specific long distance is decreased when initial muscle glycogen stores are elevated. Table 16.3 summarizes studies that have shown increased time to exhaustion related to initial muscle glycogen stores. Hermansen et al. [3] did not manipulate diets to alter initial glycogen stores yet found increased time to exhaustion related to glycogen storage. Bergstrom et al. [2] and Karlsson and Saltin [4], using two different modes of exercise, manipulated initial glycogen stores by preexercise diets. The time to exhaustion was significantly greater when cycling to exhaustion [2] and the time for a 30-km race was eight minutes faster with greater glycogen stores. When glycogen stores were doubled (1.75 g/ 100 g wet wt. versus 3.31 g/100 g wet wt.), the time to exhaustion at 80 percent $\dot{V}O_2$ max was increased from two to three hours.

Effects of Diet on Glycogen Stores

Initial glycogen stores and subsequent exercise time to exhaustion was studied by Martin et al. [9]. They found that diet was instrumental in determining preexercise glycogen stores as well as preferential use of glycogen. Work time to exhaustion at 70 percent $\dot{V}O_2$ max was more than doubled when subjects were on a high carbohydrate diet (> 75% CHO) even though the depletion phase of carbohydrate loading was not used. When a high fat/protein diet was used, only 38 percent of the energy was derived from carbohydrates whereas 72 percent of the energy came from carbohydrates with the high carbohydrate diet.

The effects of diet in a more practical sense was studied by Karlsson and Saltin [4]. Two 30-k races were preceded by either a high carbohydrate diet including the depletion phase or a mixed diet.

Table 16.3. Studies Related to Initial Glycogen Stores and Time to Exhaustion

Study	Mode	Treatment	Results

Bergstrom, Hermansen, Hultman, and Saltin, 1967	Bicycle	Preexercised diets:
		
		M = 18% P, 50% C, 30% F
		F/P –46% F, 54% P
		C = 82% C, 18% P
			Glycogen stores depleted with all diets
			
			            M F/P CHO
			Initial glycogen 1.75 .63 3.31
			(g/100 g wet wt)
			Time to exhaustion 126 59 189
			    (minus)

Karlsson and Saltin, 1971	30k race	2 diets following exercise to exhaustion: High CHO = 2500 Kcal mixed	Diet gly I gly F CHO 35g/kg 19g/kg M 17g/kg 5g/kg (30k race was 8 min. faster with CHO diet)
Hermansen, Hultman, and Saltin, 1967	Bicycle	77% $\dot{V}O_2$ max to exhaustion; trained versus untrained	Trained Untrained Initial glycogen: g/100 g wet wt. 1.6 1.6 Final glycogen: g/100 g wet wt. 1.2 .06 Time to exhaustion (min.) 90 85

They found that the carbohydrate diet resulted in twice the glycogen stores as the mixed diet. When the carbohydrate diet was used, the subjects reduced their race time by eight minutes. It was also shown by split-time analysis that the first half of the races were similar in times regardless of the diet, but that differences occurred in the second half of the race where the effects of increased carbohydrates would be most beneficial.

Bergstrom and colleagues [2,10] showed that carbohydrate replacement following exhaustion was affected by diet (Table 16.4). In a single-leg exercise to test exhaustion, they found the exercised leg almost completely depleted of glycogen while the nonexercised leg had normal glycogen stores. After one day of carbohydrate diet, the exercised leg was slightly higher in glycogen content than the nonexercised leg; following three days the exercised leg had twice the glycogen level. The control leg showed only slight increases in glycogen with diet. That diet following exhaustive exercise effects glycogen replacement was also shown in another study by Bergstrom et al. [2]. They found glycogen levels were still below preexercise levels when using a high/protein diet.

Who Should Carbohydrate Load?

On the basis of the studies reviewed, there is no doubt that carbohydrate loading is beneficial for performances that rely heavily on carbohydrates as an energy substrate. The variables to be considered include intensity, duration, muscle group involvement, and fiber recruitment patterns. In events of greater than 90 percent $\dot{V}O_2$ max, glycogen is the single most important energy substrate. During supramaximal intensity work, glycogen utilization is specific to fast twitch muscle fibers. Although concrete recommendations for carbohydrate loading for anaerobic work have not been made, it is certainly implied that workloads of 100 to 150 percent $\dot{V}O_2$ max would benefit from this practice. Maugham and Poole [14] showed that on a high carbohydrate diet the time to exhaustion at 104 percent $\dot{V}O_2$ max increased from 4.87 to 6.65 minutes while on a low carbohydrate diet the work time decreased from 4.87 minutes to 3.32 minutes. Muscle biopsy techniques were not used to determine either glycogen utilization or preferential depletion of fast twitch fibers. However, based on the Liverpool study [14] and Gollnick's et al. biopsy studies [11], one would consider the benefits of carbohydrate loading for work that relied heavily on anaerobic glycolytic pathways for energy.

Table 16.4. Studies Related to Diet and Glycogen Stores/Replacement

Study	Mode	Treatment	Results
Bergstrom and Hultman, 1966	Bicycle	One-legged exercise to exhaustion (serial biopsy) followed by 3 days of diet	Exercised leg depleted; nonexercised leg normal Day 1 of diet: exercised leg slightly more glycogen than control Day 3 of diet: exercised leg two times more glycogen stores; nonexercised leg increased slightly
Bergstrom, Hermansen, Hultman, and Saltin, 1967	Bicycle	Exercise to exhaustion	Postexercise diet of fat/protein: after 8 days glycogen still below preexercised levels. CHO diet without depletion, only moderate increased.
Karlsson and Saltin, 1971	30K run	2 races, 3 wks. apart: (1) glycogen depletion +3 days high CHO (2500 kcal) (2) glycogen depletion/mixed diet	CHO diet had two times the glycogen stores 17g versus 35 g/kg muscle Final glycogen = CHO — 19g/kg; M — 5g/kg 8 min. faster with CHO diet; split times show 1st half of race was the same, 2nd half was faster for CHO diet group
Martin et al., 1978	Treadmill 70% VO$_2$max	3 diets: (1) F/P = 90% calories (2) CHO = >75% CHO (no depletion) (3) mixed — control	F/P M CHO Work to exhaustion (mins) 33 62 77 % CHO used 1st 30 mins 38 70 72

Carbohydrate loading is beneficial for activities of 70 to 80 percent $\dot{V}O_2$ max when extended for 30 minutes or longer. The benefits vary with the diet and use of a depletion phase. Less benefit is derived by the highly trained elite athlete who typically consumes a greater carbohydrate load in order to maintain caloric balance during training.

Method of Carbohydrate Loading

Two methods are generally employed to increase muscle glycogen stores (Table 16.5). The classical method of carbohydrate loading utilizes a dietary and exercise depletion phase followed by a "loading" phase. The athletes follow a diet high in fat and protein for three to four days followed by an exhaustive run for 90 minutes. The loading phase involves three days of high carbohydrate intake with carbohydrates accounting for 75 to 90 percent of total caloric intake. It is difficult to train during the depletion phase as energy levels are progressively lowered. The athlete should not train during the loading phase because it would be counterproductive to energy storage. The classical method of carbohydrate loading should not be practiced at greater than two month intervals and should be reserved for the truly elite athlete.

The alternate method of carbohydrate loading does not result in as great a glycogen storage but is substantially easier to accomplish. The alternate method differs in that the depletion phase is not used. The loading phase should emphasize complex carbohydrates in order

Table 16.5. Techniques for Carbohydrate Loading

Days	Days Prior to Competition	Classical Method (Includes Depletion Phase)	Alternate Method (Loading Phase Only)
3–4	7	Diet high in fat and protein; only CHO to make food palatable. *Purpose*: Deplete glycogen stores.	Continue as Normally Scheduled
1	3	90 min. exhaustive run. *Purpose*: Final depletion of glycogen.	
3	3 (begin same day as exhaustive run	High complex CHO (75–90%)	High complex CHO (75–90%)

to ensure intake of essential B-complex vitamins. Simple sugars tend to suppress the appetite, and total carbohydrate intake over a three day period may be reduced when simple sugars are favored over complex carbohydrates.

FLUID REPLACEMENT

Dehydration and fluid replacement is one of the most misunderstood and misguided aspects of nutrition and performance. During exercise there is an increased fluid loss through respiration and perspiration. At rest 15 mls of water are typically lost through each respiration and perspiration. During heavy exercise water loss through respiration may increase tenfold while loss by sweating may account for 2 to 4 liters per hour period. Impairments in physical work capacity due to fluid loss has been reported by several investigators [5,6,7,8,15]. The effects of dehydration on performance is shown in Table 16.6. During exercise, water, and to a lesser extent electrolytes, is drawn from the plasma in an attempt to maintain body temperature. Acute changes in decreased plasma volume are related to water loss by sweating. Physiological changes including increased temperature, increased heart rate, and decreased stroke volume occur

Table 16.6. Dehydration Syndrome

% Plasma Volume Loss	% Body Weight	Actual Pounds (150 lb.)	Effects
2	1	1.5	Increased temperature, increased heart rate, increased thirst
4	2	3.0	
6	3	4.5	0–10% performance ⎫ normal loss
8	4	6.0	20–30% performance ⎭
10	5	7.5	Evidence of heat exhaustion
12	6	9.0	1–3% Loss Nacl 1% Loss K^+ Mg
14	7	10.5	Hallucination
16	8	12.0	Some marathoners
18	9	13.5	
20	10	15.0	Heat stroke (106–110°F) Risk of circulation collapse, convulsions

early in the dehydration syndrome. Circulation is compromised, which alternately effects the temperature control mechanisms as well as blood supply to the working muscles. There is significant interference in performance when 3 to 4 percent of the body's weight is lost in sweat.

Chronic changes in plasma volume have been studied by Costill et al. [5] who showed increased plasma volumes of 10 percent during five consecutive days of heavy work. This increased volume returned to preexercise levels following three days of inactivity. Increased plasma volume causes hemodilution and accounts for reported incidences of false anemia.

Sweat glands selectively secrete varying amounts of electrolytes by adapting to training and acclimatizing to environmental conditions. Costill [16] reports typical sodium and chloride losses of 3 to 6 percent with less than one percent potassium and magnesium loss, when total fluid loss is as high as 6 percent of body weight. It is evident that the concern for fluid loss is that of water with little concern for electrolytes. Sweat is a hypotonic solution having about one-third the concentration of Na and Cl as plasma; therefore, replacement fluids should reflect this loss.

Optimal Hydration

Optimal hydration is important to athletes engaged in endurance events but of relatively little advantage in short-term effect. Optimal hydration can be accomplished by drinking 600 mls of water (20 oz.) two hours prior to competition and another 400 to 600 mls water (14-20 oz.) 10 to 15 minutes prior to the event. From a practical point of view, the athlete is optimally hydrated when he/she must urinate frequently.

Rehydration During Performance

The greatest concern of fluid loss is that of water replacement because of its importance in preventing heat injuries and maintaining metabolic efficiency. Electrolyte and sugar intake during exercise are a secondary concern. Table 16.7 outlines the factors most important to fluid replacement. It is important to replace as much fluid as possible while not causing gastric discomfort. Costill and Saltin [17] have shown that volumes of 150 to 250 mls (5-8.5 oz.) at 10- to 15-minute intervals offer optimal fluid replacement. Fluids empty from the stomach more quickly when they are slightly cooled (41°F).

Table 16.7. Rehydration during Performance

Volume:	150–250 mls (5–8.5 oz)
Time:	10–15 mins. intervals
Temperature:	41°F
Sugar Content:	2–2.5g glucose/100 mls water (2–2.5% glucose)

Gastric distress is often misdirected to the temperature of replacement fluids when the cause is often large volumes. The most influential factor associated with gastric emptying is its glucose content. Costill and Saltin [17] report that 400 mls water will be 60 to 70 percent emptied in 15 minutes after ingestion. The same volume of soft drink containing 40 g glucose will have emptied only five percent in the same time period.

The American College of Sports Medicine [1] recommends that replacement fluids contain no more than 2 to 2.5 g of glucose per 100 mls water (2–2.5% glucose). During cold weather training and competition, there is less demand for temperature control with less fluid loss through perspiration. Because stomach emptying is less urgent, 15 to 40 percent glucose solutions are acceptable. Table 16.8 shows the suger content of popular replacement fluids. Many commercial drinks can be effectively used by diluting the product with water to meet the 2.5 percent glucose criteria.

Table 16.8. Sugar Content of Replacement Fluids (Based on Nutritional Information on Package)

Product	Glucose (g/100 mls)
A.I.D.	8.0
Competition II	1.6
Gatorade	5.6
Lasco	6.0
Pripps Pluss	6.8
Soft Drinks	10.1
ACSM	2.5
Recommendation	(15–40, cold environment)

Rehydration Following Competition

Fluid replacement during activity will not adequately replace all the fluids lost. Costill [18] found that voluntary rehydration during a 3- to 4-hour period replaced only 60 percent of the water lost during heavy work. It is estimated to take 24 to 36 hours to replace water lost during heavy work in hot, humid environments.

PREGAME/PRECOMPETITION MEALS

Pregame or precompetition means can inversely effect performance when important guidelines are not followed. It is important to realize, however, that pregame meals are not required for energy for performance. Inappropriate dietary practices will impede performance so that the athlete cannot attain the greatest benefits from condition and training. It is most important that the gastrointestinal tract is empty at the time of competition. To accomplish this, small meals of 500 kcal are suggested. The composition of the pregame meal should be low fats and fiber because those nutrients slow digestion and subsequent emptying of the GI tract. Additionally, spicy foods and foods causing gas should be avoided for obvious reasons of gastric and intestinal distress.

It is recommended that the pregame meal contain 500 kcal of complex carbohydrate and afford optimal hydration by choosing foods that are familiar to the athlete.

Many athletes are concerned with eating between events when competition continues over several hours such as in tournaments, track meets, and multiteam events. The same principles apply; at the time of competition the GI tract should be empty and the meals or snack should afford optimal hydration. To meet the unique situation, the athlete can consume low fat meals, including fruits, juices, water, light sandwiches, and the like. High-concentrated sugar snacks such as candy bars and highly sugared snacks should be consumed approximately 30 minutes prior to competition because of the insulin effect associated with them.

REFERENCES

1. American College of Sports Medicine. Position statement: Prevention of heat injuries during distance running. *Med. Sci. Sports*, 7, 1975.

2. Bergstrom, J., Hermansen, L. E., Hultman, E., and Saltin B. Diet, muscle glycogen and physical performance. *Acta Physiol. Scand.*, *71*, 140-150, 1967.

3. Hermansen, L., Hultman, E., and Saltin, B. Muscle glycogen during prolonged severe exercise. *Acta Physiol. Scand.*, *71*, 129-139, 1967.

4. Karlsson, J., and Saltin, B. Diet muscle glycogen, and endurance performance. *J. Appl. Physiol.*, *31*, 203-206, 1971.

5. Costill, D. L., and Fink, W. Plasma volume changes following exercise and thermal dehydration. *J. Appl. Physiol.*, *37*, 521-525, 1974.

6. Fink, W. J. Fluid intake for maximizing athletic performance. In W. Haskell et al. (Eds.), *Nutrition and athletic performance* (pp. 52-66). Palo Alto, CA: Bull Pub. Co., 1982.

7. Herbert, W. G., and Ribisl, P. M. Effects of dehydration upon physical work capacity of wrestlers under competitive conditions. *Res. Quart.*, *43*, 416-422, 1972.

8. Ribisl, P. M., and Herbert, W. G. Effects of rapid weight reduction and subsequent rehydration upon the physical work capacity of wrestlers. *Res. Quart.*, *41*, 536-541, 1970.

9. Martin, B., Robinson, S., and Robertshaw, D. Influence on diet on leg uptake of glucose during heavy exercise. *Am. J. Clin. Nut.*, *31*, 62-67, 1978.

10. Bergstrom, J., and Hultman, E. Muscle glycogen synthesis after exercise—An enhancing factor localized to the muscle cells in man. *Nature*, *210*, 309-310, 1966.

11. Gollnick, P. D., Armstrong, R. B., Sembrowich, W. L., Shepherd, R. E., and Saltin, B. Glycogen depletion pattern in human skeletal muscle fibers after heavy exercise. *J. Appl. Physiol.*, *34*, 615-618, 1973.

12. Havel, R. J., Naimark, A., and Borchgrevink, C. F. Turn-over rate and oxidation of free fatty acids of blood plasma in man during exercise. *J. Clin. Invest.*, *42*, 1054-1063, 1963.

13. Costill, D. L., Sparks, K., Gregar, R., and Turner, C. Muscle glycogen utilization during exhaustive running. *J. Appl. Physiol.*, *31*, 353-356, 1971.

14. Runners World, April 1982, p. 105. Citing: Maughan, R. S. and Poole, D. C., Liverpool Polytechnic Institute.

15. Costill, D. L., Cote, R., and Fink, W. Muscle water and electrolytes following varied levels of dehydration in man. *J. Appl. Physiol.*, *40*, 6-11, 1976.

16. Costill, D. L. Fluids for athletic performance: Why and what should you drink during prolonged exercise. In E. Burke (Ed.)., *Toward an understanding of human performance*. Ithaca, NY: Movement Publications, 1977.

17. Costill, D. L., and Saltin, B. Factors limiting gastric emptying during rest and exercise. *J. Appl. Physiol.*, *37*, 679-683, 1974.

18. Costill, D. L. Water and electrolytes. In W. P. Morgan (Ed.), *Ergogenic aids and muscular performance* (pp. 293-320). New York: Academic Press, 1972.

19. Costill, D. L., Branam, G., Fink, W., and Nelson, R. Exercise induced sodium conservation: Changes in plasma renin and aldosterone. *Med. Sci. Sports, 8*, 209-213, 1977.

20. Consolazio, F., and Johnson, H. L. Dietary carbohydrate and work capacity. *Am. J. Clin. Nut., 25*, 85-89, 1972.
21. Piehl, K. Glycogen storage and depletion in human skeletal muscle fibers. *Acta Physiol. Scand., 402*,(Suppl.), 1974.
22. Astrand, P. O., and Saltin, B. Plasma and red cell volume after prolonged severe exercise. *J. Appl. Physiol., 19*, 829-832, 1964.
23. Kozlowski, S., and Saltin, B. Effects of sweat loss on body fluids. *J. Appl. Physiol., 19*, 1119-1124, 1964.
24. Snellen, J. W. Body temperature during exercise. *Med. Sci. Sports, 1*, 39-42, 1969.
25. Horstman, D. H. Nutrition. In W. P. Morgan (Ed.), *Ergogenic aids and muscular performance* (pp. 343-365). New York: Academic Press, 1982.
26. Costill, D. L. Fats and carbohydrates as determinants of athletic performance. In E. Haskell et al. (Eds.), *Nutrition and athletic performance* (pp. 16-28). Palo Alto, CA: Bull Pub. Co., 1982.
27. Essen, B. Intramuscular substrate utilization during prolonged exercise. In P. Milvy (Ed.), *The marathon: Physiological, medical, epidemiological, and psychological studies* (Vol. 301, pp. 30-44). New York: New York Academy of Sciences.

Afterword

CHAPTER 17

Aerobic Capacity and the Aged Athlete

Michael L. Pollock and Thomas T. Gushiken

Recent efforts of the American Heart Association, American of Sports Medicine, and the President's Council on Physical Fitness and Sports have emphasized the need for exercise programs for all ages. Holloszy [9], in an article discussing "directions" in the area of exercise, health, and aging, wrote "Exercise provides a needed stimulus for the maintenance of structural and functional integrity of the cardiovascular system, the skeletal muscles, bones, tendons and ligaments, and probably also the autonomic nervous system and motor neurons."

More and more individuals are participating in vigorous events such as marathon runs, cross-country skiing, swimming, and cycling. The age of participants is varied and includes a large percentage of older individuals. With the keen interest of all age groups in participating in aerobic exercise, it is easy to understand an increase in participation at the Master's level (competition at 40 years of age and above).

It is generally agreed that maximal oxygen uptake ($\dot{V}O_2$ max) is the best single physiological indicator of the capacity of the respiratory and circulatory systems to supply oxygen to the working muscles and of the tissues to utilize it [2,16]. The capacities of athletes to sustain severe and sustained effort are dependent to a large extent upon the maximal rate of oxidative energy release in the working muscles, and therefore upon their $\dot{V}O_2$ max. Bruce [3] stated that "Aging is a multifactorial process which alters structures and reduces function of cells and tissues of many organs systems and $\dot{V}O_2$ is the best single variable to define the changes in functional limits of aerobic metabolism and the cardiovascular system which occurs with aging."

It has been shown that the aerobic capacity of elite endurance athletes is usually above 70 ml·kg^{-1}·min^{-1} for males and slightly lower for females [2,4,16,19,20]. The aerobic capacity of football backs, soccer players, Olympic speed skaters average in the high 50s and low 60s [11,17,21]. Healthy men above 50 years of age who exercise vigorously on a regular basis have been known to have a $\dot{V}O_2$ max 20–30% higher than that of young sedentary men [6,7,14]. Heath et al. [7] found that middle-aged and older Master's athletes who train for competition in middle and long-distance running have a $\dot{V}O_2$ max 50% or more higher than athletes of the same age who became sedentary and had stopped running when they were young. Dill [5] reported that Clarence DeMar, the famous marathon runner, at the age of 50 years has a $\dot{V}O_2$ max of 60 ml·kg^{-1}·min^{-1}. When DeMar died at age 70 of cancer, the autopsy revealed his vessels to be free from coronary atherosclerosis.

There has been difficulty in interpreting the decline in aerobic capacity found in Master's athletes. Is the decline in aerobic capacity a result of the subjects change in their quantity and quality of training? If so, the decline in aerobic capacity may be due in part to the decrease in training rather than just age in itself. It has been estimated that after maturity the reduction of aerobic capacity is approximately 9% per decade over the course of a lifetime [8]. Figure 17.1 shows the decline in $\dot{V}O_2$ max of 27 regional and national champion master's runners [14]. The decline is particularly pronounced after age 69. The data from Figure 17.1 shows a significant reduction in training miles/week with age which also parallels the reduction in aerobic capacity. This finding suggests that a reduction in aerobic capacity with age may be associated with a change in lifestyle.

The data dealing with aerobic capacity and aging most often reflect cross-sectional studies with few studies utilizing the longitudinal information on the same population. Also, often young athletes who train 100 miles per week are compared with Master's athletes who train only 20–40 miles per week. Except for the report

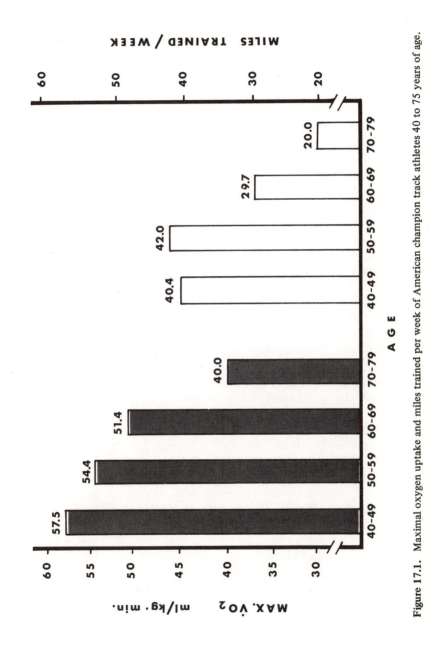

Figure 17.1. Maximal oxygen uptake and miles trained per week of American champion track athletes 40 to 75 years of age.

of Kasch and Wallace [10], the longitudinal data on non-athletes follows a similar pattern as described for athletes.

Åstrand et al. [1] studied the aerobic capacity of 66 subjects (35 female and 31 male). In 1949, the subjects were physical education students and in 1970, they were reexamined. The follow-up results revealed a 20% decline in $\dot{V}O_2$ max. During the intervening period of 21 years, the majority of subjects had been physically inactive both in their vocations and in their spare time. Robinson et al. [18] studied 37 men who were initially tested when they were healthy college students aged 18-22 years. The subjects were retested at ages 40-44 and again at ages 49-53. At ages 40-44 years, mean $\dot{V}O_2$ max had declined 25%. Eight of the men improved an average of 11% in $\dot{V}O_2$ max between ages 40-44 and 49-53 years while mean $\dot{V}O_2$ max of the others continued to decline with age. The five men who improved most had increased their participation in vigorous activities and had quit or reduced their smoking.

Heath et al. [7] compared a group of middle-aged and older endurance athletes, active in age group (Master's) competition with a group of young athletes of similar body weight. The groups were matched with regard to their habital exercise programs to avoid the confusing effects of differences in exercise training. The athletes were also compared with healthy untrained middle-aged men. The results showed that the Master's athletes were 15% lower than the young athletes in $\dot{V}O_2$ max. There was a large difference between the Master's athletes and the untrained middle-aged men (62%). The researchers hypothesized from their findings and from others [8], that if physical activity and body composition are kept constant, deterioration due to the aging process per se may result in a decline in $\dot{V}O_2$ max of only 5% per decade. Their findings also suggested that in middle-aged men who exercise vigorously on a regular basis, the major factor in the decline of $\dot{V}O_2$ max is the slowing of the maximum heart rate. Finally, the researchers concluded that despite the inevitable decrease in heart rate and $\dot{V}O_2$ max with age, some men in their sixties and seventies are able, by means of exercise training, to maintain their $\dot{V}O_2$ max above that of healthy untrained young men (see Figure 17.2).

More recently, Pollock et al. [13] completed a 10-year follow-up study on champion Master's runners. Important questions included the following: (1) Is the aging curve linear over a broad range of ages? That is, is there a continuous 9% reduction in $\dot{V}O_2$ max per decade or are the reductions more phasic? (2) If a person continues to train at the same level, will a reduction in aerobic capacity occur?

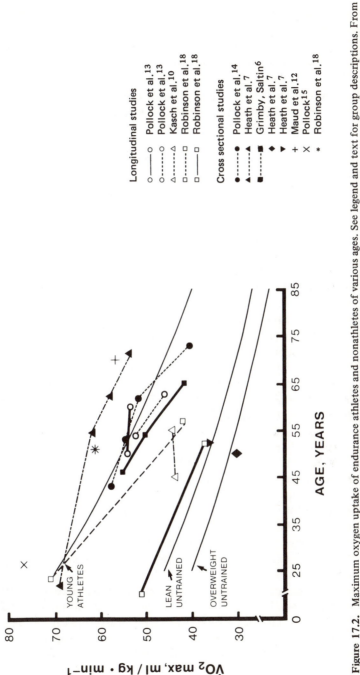

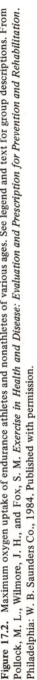

Figure 17.2. Maximum oxygen uptake of endurance athletes and nonathletes of various ages. See legend and text for group descriptions. From Pollock, M. L., Wilmore, J. H., and Fox, S. M. *Exercise in Health and Disease: Evaluation and Prescription for Prevention and Rehabilitation.* Philadelphia: W. B. Saunders Co., 1984. Published with permission.

The cross-sectional results from this group's 1971 data showed the expected decrease in $\dot{V}O_2$ max up to approximately 65 years of age, with a more dramatic reduction occurring thereafter (see Figure 17.1). As a result of the small sample studied who were older than the age of 70 and the significant difference in the quantity and quality of training among the various age groups, conclusions were considered somewhat tenuous. Was the reduction in aerobic capacity a result of aging or the difference in training level?

The follow-up data were collected on 25 men 50–82 years of age. All of the subjects had continued their training but only 11 were training at approximately the same level and were still highly competitive. Training mileage remained unchanged for both groups, but the post-competitors slowed their training pace by approximately 2 minutes per mile. Figure 17.1 shows the results in $\dot{V}O_2$ max. The competitive group showed no significant change in $\dot{V}O_2$ max (54.2 versus 53.3 ml $\cdot$ kg^{-1} $\cdot$ min^{-1}), whereas the post-competitive group decreased significantly (52.5 versus 45.9 ml $\cdot$ kg^{-1} $\cdot$ min^{-1}). The post-competitive group's decrease in $\dot{V}O_2$ max followed the expected aging curves. The results of this study help to confirm the hypothesis that the reduction in aerobic capacity found with age is affected by maintenance of training. This hypothesis is in agreement with the previously mentioned results of Kasch and Wallace [10]. The data also showed the aging curve for aerobic capacity to be curvilinear rather than linear, as reported by other research [7,8]. The competitive group who continued to train at the same intensity level showed no reduction in $\dot{V}O_2$ max until after age 60 to 65 years. After this age, a decrease was evident but not at the same rate as shown in the cross-sectional studies. Although the longitudinal studies of Kasch and Wallace [10] and Pollock et al. [13] seem to answer important questions about how exercise may affect cardio-respiratory fitness with age, more data using larger numbers of subjects and longer follow-up periods are necessary before final conclusions can be drawn.

In summary, the older endurance athlete has a significantly higher aerobic capacity than his/her sedentary counterpart. This difference is illustrated in Figure 17.2. Although both active and sedentary men and women show an average 9% reduction in $\dot{V}O_2$ max per decade of life, much of this reduction may be affected by reduced training. More recent data on Master's athletes as well as nonathletes suggest that the reduction in aerobic capacity to be less than 5% per decade for persons who remain highly active.

REFERENCES

1. Åstrand, I., Åstrand, P. O., Hallback, I., and Kilbom, A. Reduction in maximal oxygen uptake with age. *J. Appl. Physiol. 35*, 649–654, 1973.
2. Åstrand, P. O., and Rodahl, K. *Textbook of Work Physiology*, 2nd ed. New York: McGraw-Hill Book Co., 1977.
3. Bruce, R. A. Exercise, functional aerobic capacity, and aging—another viewpoint. *Med. Sci. Sports Exerc. 16*, 8–13, 1984.
4. Costill, D. L. The Physiology of Marathon Running. *JAMA. 221*, 1024–1029, 1972.
5. Dill, D. B. Marathoner DeMar: Physiological studies. *J. Nat. Cancer Inst. 35*, 185–191, 1965.
6. Grimby, G., and Saltin, B. Physiological analysis of physically well-trained middle-aged and old athletes. *Acta Med. Scand. 179*, 513–525, 1966.
7. Heath, G. W., Hagberg, J. M., Ehsani, A. A., and Holloszy, J. O. A physiological comparison of young and older endurance athletes. *J. Appl. Physiol. 51*, 634–640, 1981.
8. Hodgson, J. L., and Buskirk, E. R. Physical fitness and age, with emphasis on cardiovascular function in the elderly. *J. Amer. Geriatr. Soc. 25*, 385–392, 1977.
9. Holloszy, J. O. Exercise, health and aging: a need for more information. *Med. Sci. Sports Exerc. 15*, 1–5, 1983.
10. Kasch, F., and Wallace, J. P. Physiological variables during 10 years of endurance exercise. *Med. Sci. Sports 8*, 5–8, 1976.
11. Maksud, M. G., Farrell, P., Foster, C., Pollock, M. L., Anholm, J., Hare, J., and Schmidt, D. Maximal $\dot{V}O_2$ max, ventilation, and heart rate of Olympic speed skating candidates. *J. Sports Med. 22*, 217–223, 1982.
12. Maud, P. J., Pollock, M. L., Foster, C., Anholm, J., Gutton, G., Al-Nouri, M., Hellman, C., and Schmidt, D. H. Fifty years of training and competition in the marathon: Wally Hayward aged 70—a physiological profile. *S. Afr. Med. J. 59*, 153–157, 1981.
13. Pollock, M. L., Foster, C., Rod, J., Hare, J., and Schmidt, D. H. Ten year follow-up on the aerobic capacity of champion master's track athletes. *Med. Sci. Sports Exer. 14*, 105, 1982.
14. Pollock, M. L., Miller, H. S., and Wilmore, J. Physiological characteristics of champion American track athletes 40–75 years of age. *J. Gerontol. 29*, 645–649, 1974.
15. Pollock, M. L. Submaximal and maximal working capacity of elite distance runners. *Ann. N. Y. Acad. Sci. 301*, 310–322, 1977.
16. Pollock, M. L., Wilmore, J. H., and Fox, S. M. *Exercise in Health and Disease: Evaluation and Prescription for Prevention and Rehabilitation.* Philadelphia: W. B. Saunders Co., 1984.
17. Raven, P. B., Gettman, L. R., Pollock, M. L., and Cooper, K. H. A physiological evaluation of professional soccer players. *Brit. J. Sports Med. 10*, 209–216, 1976.

18. Robinson, S., Dill, D. B., Tzankoff, S. P., Wagner, J. A., and Robinson, R. D. Longitudinal studies of aging in 37 men. *J. Appl. Physiol. 38*, 263–267, 1975.
19. Vaccaro, P., Morris, A. F., and Clarke, D. H. Physiological characteristics of master's female distance runners. *Phys. Sports Med. 9*, 105-108, 1981.
20. Wilmore, J. H., and Brown, C. H. Physiological profile of women distance runners. *Med. Sci. Sports 6*, 178-181, 1974.
21. Wilmore, J. H., and Haskell, W. Body composition and endurance capacity of professional football players. *J. Appl. Physiol. 33*, 564-567, 1972.

Index